The Marshall Plan:

Being Good to Be Bad

It's not a diet. It's a lifestyle.

Cindi Marshall Oakey

BALBOA.
PRESS
A DIVISION OF HAY HOUSE

Balboa Press books may be ordered through booksellers or by contacting:

Balboa Press
A Division of Hay House
1663 Liberty Drive
Bloomington, IN 47403
www.balboapress.com
1-(877) 407-4847

Because of the dynamic nature of the Internet, any web addresses or
links contained in this book may have changed since publication and
may no longer be valid. The views expressed in this work are solely those
of the author and do not necessarily reflect the views of the publisher,
and the publisher hereby disclaims any responsibility for them.

The author of this book does not dispense medical advice or prescribe the use
of any technique as a form of treatment for physical, emotional, or medical
problems without the advice of a physician, either directly or indirectly. The
intent of the author is only to offer information of a general nature to help you
in your quest for emotional and spiritual well-being. In the event you use any
of the information in this book for yourself, which is your constitutional right,
the author and the publisher assume no responsibility for your actions.

Any people depicted in stock imagery provided by Thinkstock are models,
and such images are being used for illustrative purposes only.
Certain stock imagery © Thinkstock.

Printed in the United States of America.

ISBN: 978-1-4525-7467-7 (sc)
ISBN: 978-1-4525-7468-4 (e)

Library of Congress Control Number: 2013909438

Balboa Press rev. date: 06/21/13

This book is dedicated to my mom and dad
for instilling the values in me that make it all possible.

TABLE OF CONTENTS

FORWARD

I STARTED WRITING this book over fifteen years ago. I originally called it, The Marshall Plan: The Party Girl's Guide to Eat, Drink, & Stay Slim, but I'm no longer a party girl. However, I do love to eat really good food, socialize with a cocktail or two (or three...), and I'm forever trying to stay in my skinny jeans.

I had been a lifelong serial dieter, trying all the fads throughout the 1980s and 90s. I realized that wasn't working any more and, in more recent years I've become a certified Health Coach, learning about nutritional value and a more wholesome way of eating for better health and vitality, and shedding a few pounds to get back into my skinny jeans.

The Marshall Plan: Being Good to Be Bad is a compilation of my years of trying this and trying that, gaining knowledge and expertise along the way. It's not a diet, it's a lifestyle change. There are no hard and fast rules. Once you know the ins and outs, you decide what you want to eat. You'll know the healthy choices, and you'll have the knowledge you need to choose when to Be Good and when to splurge and Be Bad. And you'll know that Being Bad is a treat, not the norm.

I repeat myself throughout the book – intentionally. Sometimes I repeat myself to drive home a point. In other cases I repeat myself because the foundational principles overlap from one category to another. As we know, we learn through repetition.

The Marshall Plan is a lifestyle change, not a diet.

At some point in life, man or woman, the age thing catches up to us. What we always did to stay slim doesn't work any more.

The Marshall Plan is a shift for healthy-minded people who have come to the realization that what they always did to stay fit, trim, and looking good isn't working anymore. It's especially for you if, like most people I know, you enjoy good food and a libation (or two, or three, or....)

That's why I say that The Marshall Plan a lifestyle change, not a diet. Following The Marshall Plan will be *relatively* easy if you're a woman who wants to lose five to ten pounds, or less than 10% of your current weight. It will also be *relatively* easy if you're a man who wants to lose ten to twenty pounds. I say *relatively* easy because it's never *really* easy, and you have to seriously want results in order to achieve results.

We'll talk about ideal eating strategies, yet the best part of The Marshall Plan is that there's no expectation to strictly enforce all the rules all the time. That wouldn't be fun, nor would it be realistically feasible.

The Marshall Plan is more of a sliding scale than a rulebook or diet book. There are no meal plans, but there are recommended foods to eat and foods to stay away from. You get to decide which guidelines to adopt and how often.

As you begin to see results, you may be inspired to follow the guidelines more often. Or you may reach your goals and boomerang back to old habits. Or a one-week vacation could throw the whole plan off.

The good news is that you'll always have the tools to get back on track, however gradual or strict you choose to be. It's a lifestyle change that doesn't happen overnight, but as you gradually learn more about making smart choices it will become life-long.

Throughout this book I refer to eating in an ideal world: eating whole, fresh foods that are closest to their most natural state. When you understand the meaning of the *ideal* world, you'll learn how to make smarter choices when you're faced with *real* world options, good or bad. That's why I also often refer to some fast food options, but "fast food" doesn't mean McDonald's, Wendy's, or Moe's. When I say "fast food," I mean foods that are quickly available when you're in a hurry or dining out.

Making The Marshall Plan's lifestyle change allows you to choose your guilt free splurges, and will help you know when you need to pull back so as not to sabotage your weight goals – or, as I like to put it, to stay comfortable in your skinny jeans.

If you feel that you need to lose more than 10 to 20 percent of your body weight, you most likely need a more structured diet program. If that's the case, consult your health practitioner to determine a program that's right for you. That said, my professional opinion (not a paid endorsement) is that Weight Watchers is the most natural program that can help you learn to make smart choices, altering your current eating habits and helping you lose weight.

In both schools of thought, The Marshall Plan or Weight Watchers, you learn to make choices that support your goal to look good at a lower weight. It's not about depriving yourself. When you deprive yourself it gets very difficult to stick to a plan. If you eat good, satisfying food daily, you can gradually lose weight, and you can learn to maintain your weight within your goal range.

I understand what it means to struggle with the conflicts between weight, healthy eating, and the compelling desire to have fun.

A very bright colleague once asked me, "How do I know you're not just a skinny bitch drinking a beer?"

Many people don't know that I've struggled with my weight since high school, easily gaining weight from overeating. In high school, extracurricular activities like cheerleading and running track burned off the chocolate and peanut butter rice krispy treats I ate for lunch and the Doritos and Tab I had after school.

It all came to a screeching halt after graduation when I went to an eight-to-five desk job. By Thanksgiving when the gang got together for the annual Turkey Bowl (bowling alley after family dinner), I cried when a friend asked why I was wearing a denim skirt to go bowling. My jeans were too tight.

That holiday season an even sadder behavior reared its ugly head: bulimia. I didn't know the word until

Princess Diana brought it to the media's attention nearly fifteen years later, but I took medication to vomit after over-eating at one holiday party so I could pig out at a second party that same evening. Needless to say I spent the night hugging the porcelain throne, and it wasn't fun.

Learned Behavior

I dedicate this book to my mother.

In her own way, she fought her Italian family's genetic disposition to be overweight.

Her older sister was obese. My mother, her younger sister, and my grandmother were petite women with fireplug silhouettes: large breasts, wide waist and belly, full hips and thighs.

Since the 1960s I remember my 5'3" mother, a size 4, 6, or 8, eating cottage cheese and canned fruit, a half a grapefruit, or a plain hamburger patty. My guess is that she was hungry much of the time.

I remembered what she ate and what she didn't eat, and I heard her talk anxiously about "getting fat." I learned that dieting and deprivation were a solution to prevent getting fat, and the roller coaster began.

I fought overeating and binge dieting for the next thirty-plus years until I learned to eat fresh, whole food. Even today, I cannot have a bag of cookies, candy, or snacks around the house because I will devour them. The best way for me to exert self-control is to not have treats in the house and only eat them when dining out, making the conscious choice to do so.

Over the years, I've used what I learned through experience and study to refine my "Marshall Plan" Being Good to Be Bad. More recently, I've incorporated my studies in nutrition and what it really means to eat well into The Plan. I've learned for myself and for my clients that it's possible to eat yummy, nutrient-dense foods, cut back on hidden sugars, and enjoy yourself. It's not all steamed broccoli and plain grilled chicken!

The final piece fell into place for me when I studied at the Institute of Integrative Nutrition where I learned about what's called Primary Foods – relationships, career, spirituality – the aspects of life that create joy and inspiration.

Looking back, it's easy for me to see that the times when my weight was most out of control were those times when the primary foods in my life were most out of balance.

I truly believe that when we're tuned in, aware of our feelings and emotions, we can rise above the doldrums. Knowledge is power, and as individuals we can take power in our own happiness – and in our own healthy choices.

The focus of this program is to learn to eat more whole food when given the opportunity. There are several contemporary terms that are often used define whole foods. An easy way to remember the meaning is with the acronym SLOW: Seasonal, Local, Organic, and Whole.

According to Wikipedia, **whole foods** are foods that are unprocessed and unrefined, or processed and refined as little as possible, before being consumed. Whole foods typically do not contain added ingredients such as salt, carbohydrates, or fats. Examples of whole foods include unpolished grains, beans, fruits, vegetables, and non-homogenized dairy products. (We won't go there since one goal is to reduce and choose dairy wisely.)

Also according to Wikipedia, the international **Slow Food movement** was founded by Carlo Petrini in 1986. Promoted as an alternative to fast food, it strives to preserve traditional and regional cuisine and encourages farming of plants, seeds, and livestock characteristic of the local ecosystem. The goal is to promote sustainable foods and local small business, working against the trend towards globalization of agriculture..

A **locavore** is a person interested in eating food that's locally produced rather than moved long distances to market. The locavore movement grew out of an increasing interest in sustainability and eco-consciousness. The food may be grown in home gardens or by local commercial groups interested in keeping the environment as clean as possible, selling food close to where it is grown. One definition of "local" food is food grown within 100 miles of its point of purchase or consumption.

All these terms define perspectives that can help you think about the choices you make. This being said, throughout this book there will be a few recommendations for when you're on the go that rely on prepared foods that aren't necessarily in their most natural state. That's because we don't live in a perfect world or have a personal chef to shop and prepare food for us every day. You need to know smart choices when you're on the go or in hurry.

Overall, the main goal is to make the most **nutrient dense** choices whenever possible.

CHAPTER 1

Getting Started

THERE ARE NO finite rules in eating healthy. The Marshall Plan is a lifestyle change that teaches and subsequently allows you to make smart choices. Since there are no finite rules, you may read parts of The Plan and think, I've heard different, and most likely you have. The following theories have worked for me and many of my health coaching clients, and are adopted from the lessons I learned while becoming a certified health coach. When in doubt, you should *always check with your health practitioner* for what is best for your dietary needs.

First and foremost, don't tell people you're on a diet. Remember, you're changing your eating habits and creating a new lifestyle approach to food and weight.

Do you think you know what to eat, what's healthy and what's not? You're reading this because you want to make a change, so I ask you to be open-minded about new ideas. I'm fascinated when I overhear intelligent people discuss old-school thoughts about food and diet – ideas that they're taking out of context and ideas that are just plain foolish.

The truth is that no one eating plan works for everyone. The Marshall Plan is about eating, drinking, and looking good, not about rigidity. It's about finding a balance of making healthier choices, and choosing guilt free splurges wisely. *You* get to plan how *you* want to orchestrate your eating habits. That's a big responsibility, so the more you know about different eating philosophies, the more diverse your choices can be.

In an ideal world, we could eat organic, fresh, yummy foods all the time, but the reality is we don't always have that option. We have to learn how to adapt to highs and lows in life, emotional challenges as well as happy times, holidays, family, and dirty-little-secret guilty food desires. All these and more influence our triggers for healthy and unhealthy eating choices. In The Marshall Plan, you decide when to splurge and how you'll compensate for those splurges. I call it "**Being Good to Be Bad**."

One of my most successful lifelong philosophies for maintaining weight (my real goal is to stay in my current jeans size) is Being Good to Be Bad. It allows me to stabilize my eating habits so I don't feel deprived, and allows me to eat almost everything I desire, even if not as often as I'd like, and always taking quantity into consideration. Mostly Being Good to Be Bad means eating healthy during the week so I can splurge a little on the weekend.

This philosophy is beneficial for every situation: approaching the holiday season, your birthday, spring vacation, summertime partying, or autumn football season. Being Good to Be Bad is a key year-round tactic to eat, drink, and look good.

Being Good to Be Bad means you amp up healthier eating choices and cut back on a the splurges. Notice that I didn't say give up all splurges.

Throughout this book we'll identify what makes a good choice, and we'll identify the difference between bad choices and guilt free splurges. Once you learn the difference, you'll become aware of how often you eat things that sabotage your good intentions for healthy eating. We all play wicked mind games that enable us to conveniently forget what we consume each day. But Being Good to Be Bad means you intentionally choose good foods most of the time. It also means that you intentionally choose when to splurge on bad foods, and you enjoy your splurges to the fullest extent.

If you practice mindful eating every week, you *will* lose weight and be able to maintain your desired weight goals. You might even surprise yourself. This philosophy gets easier year after year, so as you refine your tastebuds, you might stair-step your weight down over the long haul, and you'll certainly be able to maintain your weight.

Even if you go on a week long vacation, eat and drink to your heart's content and gain five pounds, you won't panic, because by the time you've finished reading this book you'll know the tools to get back on track – and back into your skinny jeans in no time.

Quick take-away:
It's not a diet, it's a lifestyle change.

CHAPTER 2

Being Good to Be Bad

THE PHILOSOPHY OF Being Good to Be Bad starts by breaking down your weekly schedule.

You choose to Be Good on Monday through Wednesday or Thursday, depending on your social calendar. Then you can enjoy weekend meals, whether dining in or out, and make smart choices without being too rigid.

This is an ideal strategy if your goal is to maintain your weight. If you're trying to lose five pounds or more you'll have to be a little more good (while still eating and drinking.) We'll discuss these tactics later in this chapter.

In an ideal world, Being Good means:
- Choosing lean protein;
- Incorporating green vegetables in all your meals and snacks;
- Eliminating refined carbohydrates;
- Choosing whole grains;
- Reducing dairy; and

- Super-sleuthing for hidden sugars.

Let's be real: you're not going to be that good all the time. It's a goal, a parameter, a point of measure, and a little more serious than just a guideline.

The most important principle in The Marshal Plan is *ya gotta live*. Eating is an important part of living. You're learning to choose food wisely to support your good health intentions.

So what does the ideal world look like?

In an ideal world, you always choose lean protein: grilled, baked, or poached (yeah, poached is *really* being good) seafood, white meat poultry or pork, steak, or tofu. Sautéing lean protein adds flavor and is another good option. You'll learn more about specific lean protein in the coming chapters.

When you look at your plate, 30% should be lean protein and the remaining 70% as many green vegetables as you want with your meals. Your veggies can be cooked tasty as well. If you want to Be really Good, you can eat them raw or steamed, but that isn't very satisfying and doesn't last long. Try it one or two nights a week. Again, you'll learn more about types of green veggies so you can mix it up, as we know variety is the spice of life.

Throughout this book we will talk about ways to diversify your choices in all the categories. Keep that in mind, because diversity makes maintaining healthy choices easier, and becomes a way of life. You are actually training your tastebuds.

Now, when I say green veggies, I mean green veggies

for as many meals and snacks as you choose. Choose water-based vegetables instead of starchy vegetables. This means such things as colored peppers, mushrooms, and jicama are included among the more common green veggie mix.

Avocados are a good source of protein but are calorie-packed, as are edamame and legumes, so be mindful of portion sizes. We're talking about no more than a quarter of an avocado and roughly less than a half cup of legumes as a serving size. Have I been starving and eaten half an avocado? Yeah, sure. Just not most of the time, and I always make it a conscious choice.

Cut out all white processed carbs and keep whole-grain carbs to a minimum. Include small portions of less than half a cup of complex carbs in only one or two meals a day. Whole grains like quinoa, barley, brown rice, millet, spelt, or kamut are good choices to try. Don't be afraid of these less-than-familiar, nutrient-dense grains. They are available in easy to prepare packages just like nutrient-empty, wasted-calorie white rice. It's easy to experiment with different varieties of grains at the prepared food section at stores such as Whole Foods. Then you can try your own recipes if you're so inclined.

Baked sweet potatoes are a good choice, and are packed with antioxidants and nutrients – but skip the butter and sour cream. Instead, try cinnamon, a highly antioxidant spice, if you like it. I love a dollop of low-fat cottage cheese (a childhood favorite food), so I might have that on a baked sweet potato once every few months.

When limiting carbohydrates it's really, really, really important to remember that vegetables are carbohydrates, so you're not depriving yourself of this food group. I don't understand why this concept isn't more common knowledge in our society. It makes a huge difference in your success in losing or maintaining weight.

Fresh fruit is good too. Fresh fruit in the morning as it is easy to digest. Again, diversifying your fruit choices is really important because you get different vitamins from different fruits and veggies as well. You wouldn't want to eat as many fruits and veggies as needed to get your daily requirements, but mixing up your intake doesn't hurt.

Fruit is also a great snack, especially as a replacement for sweets like cookies, cakes, or candy. Having a sweet craving? Pop a handful of blueberries, or try a tangerine or clementine. Bananas and apples travel well. Stay away from or severely limit dried fruits. Craving something sweet after dinner? Try a raspberry herbal tea. Yes, that's Being *really* Good, but snacking should be eliminated after dinner. Herbal tea should be the only thing you consume after dinner when you're Being Good.

Being *really* Good? Eliminate or reduce dairy to just one or two days per week. That means limiting low fat milk, cottage cheese, and yogurt, in addition to the regular-fat cheese you've already eliminated because regular-fat dairy isn't part of Being Good. Ice cream is a splurge, yet some frozen yogurts are a good substitute *occasionally*. Later on you'll learn to read labels to determine which frozen yogurts are better choices.

Choose healthy snacks so you're never starving. Learn

to like low-sodium V8. I say "learn to like" because it's not my personal favorite thing, but it's nutrient-dense and filling, so stock the fridge. I like to down one before going out to dinner on weekends because then I stay away from the bread basket. And that reminds me: it's okay to just say "no" when the bread basket arrives at the table – especially when you're being good.

Now is the perfect time to point out that this is not a life sentence. It's temporary. You want the bread? Go for it, especially if it looks delicious, just not all the time. But wait – I've jumped ahead! We're still Being Good on Monday through Wednesday or Thursday.

Dry nights, a.k.a. no alcohol, is best while Being Good, especially at home. If you can have just one, go for it, but in my circle, we rarely just have one. Alcohol is empty calories, but 100 calories of clear liquids won't destroy the entire plan. However, beware: a little buzz can lead to overeating, whether healthy foods or splurging, and overeating defeats the purpose you're saving up for – Being Good to Be Bad.

Also, it doesn't hurt to give your organs a break from processing alcohol. If you can do without alcohol during the weeknights, 100 calories less each night means weight loss.

Of course, endless glasses of water throughout the day are essential.

Being Bad on the weekends is flexible. How Bad do you want to Be?

If you can continue to make smart choices over the weekend, you're ahead of your game and more likely to shed a few pounds. If your goal is to maintain your weight, and you lose a pound or two Monday through Wednesday or Thursday, then you won't mind if you gain a pound or two on the weekend, and it's easy to do.

Smart choices means still choosing lean meat, poultry, or seafood, and plenty of vegetables. The catch is that when you dine out you don't have as much control over the hidden ingredients used by artsy, gourmet chefs.

While it's okay to ask for special treatment, such as omitting sauces or extra salt, it's best to be selective of your changes so you aren't asking the chef to rework the entire dish. Also, on a busy night, a restaurant kitchen can only handle so many changes.

It's okay to taste the saucy flavors in a limited way, especially if you're trying to maintain, not lose, weight. Request sauce on the side so you can distribute it yourself. If that's not an option and you get an entree swimming in buttery or cheesy sauces, ask for a second plate and transfer your food to the clean plate as sauce-free as possible.

A weekend gathering often means whooping it up for a lot of people. Enjoy yourself!

Especially during the holiday season, Being Good to Be Bad becomes more difficult because social events pop up during the week as well as on the weekend.

Make your choices wisely. Birthday celebrations? Enjoy your favorite dish. Vacation? Have a frozen daiquiri. In France? Savor a croissant – daily even.

But stay sane. During football season try not to eat an entire bag of chips each day during both college games and NFL Sunday games. Can you switch to baked chips? If not, enjoy the real thing. For English football, a.k.a. soccer, we like Guinness and hand-cut chips and, we go for it; just not every weekend.

We used to love bread pudding in autumn. We don't do that anymore. Throughout the year we love a good cheese plate, but only once a month. Unless you're trying to be a swimsuit model or professional body builder, enjoy food, but don't go overboard. If you eat french fries five days a week now, can you only eat them two or three days a week instead? I'm being way too kind. Anyway, you get the idea. Be more Good than Bad each week.

One October, I had the good fortune to go to Italy for a week. Knowing my anti-carb eating habits, many friends said, "Eat the pasta!" For the record, I ate pasta and at the time, no, I had not seen the movie or read the book, *Eat, Pray, Love*, but was acutely aware of the concept. (Personally I don't believe such extreme measures are necessary, but it made her millions of dollars so yay for her.)

But here's the surprise: after a few days of pasta, I really craved green vegetables. You can train your brain.

In Italy, during three days of group meetings with limited food choices, I politely ate what was served (and I don't eat red meat.) This was mainly assorted Italian "hams," pasta with mushrooms, gnocchi with mushrooms, and I passed on medallions of beef with more mushrooms. Obviously, mushrooms were in season.

By the time we were on our own, I was craving GREEN food, which I ordered, along with grilled fish, at every opportunity. My body craved healthier choices of lean protein and green vegetables. You might say that in this situation, I was bad and then good. Of course the week prior to travel I tried to be extra good, knowing I was going to eat pasta and oh, the fresh baked bread on every table; no butter required – yum.

If you're trying to keep your weight down, you want to be more mindful of what and how you order when dining out. It's a great motivation for Being Good to Be Bad, and over the course of time, it becomes a way of life. It really works!

Quick Take-away:
Being Good to Be Bad is the secret to success.
And ya gotta Be Good more than Bad.

Being Good to Be Bad *when you want to lose 5+ pounds*

It should come to no surprise that if you want to lose weight, you have to Be more Good than Bad to achieve your goal.

This does not mean you give up all splurges. You just choose your splurges more wisely and make sure they're fewer and farther between to get the goal rolling.

With the Monday through Thursday strategy, you can stair-step your weight down over the course of a month or two. If you can lose two pounds during the weekdays, and only gain one pound on the weekend, you net a one pound loss that entire week. It takes time, but you're not dieting; you're changing your eating habits so you can maintain your desired goal, Being Good to Be Bad.

To lose 5+ pounds, you really have to eat clean foods: lean proteins at most meals with green vegetables and fresh fruit. Consider having one vegetarian meal per day, perhaps in the evening when low energy is an asset in the hours before bedtime.

Eliminate processed carbohydrates and dairy, with the exception of a rare special splurge (note: singular splurge, not plural splurges). Think WHOLE FOODS - not the grocery store, but fresh foods as close as possible to their most natural state. Whole foods are foods that come from plants, not foods that are made in plants.

How clean you eat is directly related to how fast you will achieve your goal. It really is best to change your lifestyle moderately, *yet* people can be more motivated when they *see results* on the scale or in how their pants fit.

Movement is key to burning calories and increasing your metabolism. Ideally, you already have a movement or exercise strategy as part your life. Yet for many of us what use to work no longer works, leading to weight gain, and then your jeans don't fit, and that's why you're reading this book.

If you don't already have a movement strategy in

your life, consider hiring a fitness or health coach to build your strategy. We'll talk about specifics in more detail later on.

Can you bump up your movement strategy by walking an extra 10 -15 minutes a day, maybe just two or three days a week to start? Typically, a relatively healthy person can walk a mile in 15-17 minutes. The amount of time nor the distance is not really the point. If you intentionally add more movement to your life, you will see benefits.

When you drive to the grocery store or mall, park far away rather than circling to find the nearest parking space. You'll get exercise *and* save time and stress from driving around.

One of my clients, an occasional marathon runner and mother of two young boys, wanted to lose five or six pounds before a 10-day holiday in France. I asked her if once in a while she could go out for a 20 to 30 minute run in the morning before going to work (normally, she'd run 45 to 60 minutes or not at all). She said, "Yes I can. My husband is not traveling this week, and I can ask him to get the kids up." Thrilled by her "aha" moment, she freed herself from the obligation of long runs versus not running at all.

The same holds true for walking. A short walk is better than not walking at all. If you're traveling for business, you may not want to pack workout shoes, but most likely you have shoes you can walk ten minutes one way, and ten minutes back to your hotel. You might find time to do this a few times per day, rather than carving out 45 minutes or more for a full workout.

During the crunch time before my client's holiday to France, we came up with a "Guerrilla Tactics Week" plan. This is for the do-or-die time before going on vacation or a special event. You want to loose weight. You know you need to bump up your exercise by adding 15 to 20 minute walks to your current cardio schedule. Add in other successful moves like dropping down for a 60 second plank and then side plank for 30 seconds each side. Repeat as often as possible. Can you do ten push ups when you get out of bed each morning? Ten squats while you brush your teeth? Can you increase the numbers by two each day, every few days, or each week? Create index cards as reminders and set them out so you don't forget.

It works, but there's no magic. Ya gotta Be Good to Be Bad, otherwise you have an even tougher challenge when you come home and realize your weight gain has gone too far.

Being Good to Be Bad also holds true if you want to stair-step your weight down before the holiday season kicks in so you can enjoy social gatherings more and still maintain some sort of balance during the holiday season. The goal is to Be Good whenever you can so you don't lose it, going to hell in a hand-basket and waking up miserable on January First with an unpleasantly huge goal to tackle.

Deprivation is not part of a healthy lifestyle. If you tell yourself you can never have a piece of cake, cheese, pizza, margaritas - whatever whets your whistle - you'll be unhappy and more likely to over-indulge. And we know over-indulgence leads to tight pants, and that's not fun.

The philosophy behind Being Good to Be Bad coincides with the 90/10 Diet – eat smart/healthy 90% of the time, and eat whatever you want 10% of the time. Be wary of being good 100% of the time, because that can lead to severe splurges and even bingeing. Besides, unless you live on a mountain top, who could be good 100% of the time?

It's a lifestyle change, not a diet. It takes mindful practice as in developing any skill. Like my dear friend Sarah said, "You can do it, if you really want to." That was a catalyst that lead me to lose over 12 pounds over the course of three years, and start writing this book again.

Quick take-away:
Being Good to Be Bad is the secret to success. And ya gotta Be extra Good to lose a few pounds before you can Be Bad.

CHAPTER 3

Just Say No

EARLIER, I SAID The Marshall Plan was *relatively* easy, yet it wasn't going to be *really* easy. There are some things that you shouldn't eat unless you are making a cognitive choice to Be Bad. This means that when you are Being Good, you have to learn to Just Say No.

Remember, this is not a life sentence; this is to get started. Once you achieve your goals, you can add treats into your eating plan. But be wary – for some of us, just a few days or a week of not paying attention can mean two to five extra pounds and painfully tight jeans.

So The Marshall Plan begins with one simple direction, Just Say No to the list of foods and beverages below.

Some of you might ask why these items are "no" items. As a child, my father had just one answer to that question. "Because I said so," he'd say with a smile. With the utmost respect for my father, the philosophy in The Marshall Plan reflects the same directive.

I'm kidding ...but not really. As we go forward in specific chapters, you'll gain insight into the answers as to "why?" so you can make your own smart choices once you've reached your desired goal. You're not expected to never eat these foods again. You Just Say No to get started so you begin to see results. Results motivate you on the path to success.

Your success is based on a balance of lean protein, monounsaturated and healthy polyunsaturated fats, and whole grain carbohydrates. Again, think fresh whole foods versus manufactured and processed foods.

Remember, this is a temporary strategy, not a life sentence. Once you begin to see results, you can include your favorite foods in moderation.

- No soda, no diet soda, no fruit juices.
- No fried foods.
- No butter, no mayonnaise, no ketchup, no BBQ sauce, no mustard.
- No white potatoes: baked, mashed, fries, or chips. Boiled new potatoes or baked sweet potatoes are acceptable if your goals are moderate, 1x / week, or aggressive, 1 x / month. Roasted new or sweet potatoes should be limited, but if your goals are moderate you can have them 1 x / week, versus aggressive, 1x / month.
- No white rice or pilaf.
- No grits, for my friends in the south.
- No white flour pasta.
- No white bread, rolls, bagels, focaccia, croissants, muffins, sweet rolls, and need I say cinnamon buns? If you want a burger or a sandwich, eat just one piece of bread; eat it open-faced.

- No sugary cereals. Beware of boxes labeled "whole grain." They can be deceptive.
- No granola.
- No soup in restaurants; they tend to contain mysterious bad fat.
- No cheddar, Swiss, Colby, jack, pepper jack cheese on sandwiches, salads* or in main dishes like chicken or fish. Dry cheeses like feta, ricotta, gorgonzola, parmesan, asiago, part-skim mozzarella, and goat cheese are better choices in moderation.
- No buttery or creamy sauces. When dining out, either order sauce on the side or transfer your meat and veggies to a separate small plate such as a bread plate – which will be clean since you're not eating bread.
- No fruit-on-the-bottom yogurt or yogurt smoothie drinks.
- No alcohol during the week at home. If you're out with friends on a weekday, drink one or two glasses of white wine, vodka soda w/ lemon or lime, or light beer.
- No EATING ANYTHING AFTER 8pm.

To get started, pick a goal: let's say for one month, you'll Just Say No to the foods on the list. You might find having a conversation with yourself, either in your head or out loud if necessary, will help remind you that these foods will be available another time in life, once you've met your goals. Then, you can make a cognitive choice when to enjoy them.

Depending on your desired weight-loss goal, or whether you want to maintain your current weight, you can exercise the greatest restraint Monday through Thursday, and either be totally free on the weekends or conscientiously moderate.

So what can you eat you ask, sniff, sniff? We'll start talking about specifics in the next chapter.

Quick take-away:
If you want to be slim, ya gotta Be Good much of the time. Ya gotta learn to Just Say No.

CHAPTER 4

Vegetables and Fruits

VEGETABLES OR FRUITS should make up fifty percent of every meal. Funny how we've heard this all our lives and it comes back full circle.

There's a huge difference now from when most of us were kids because we have access to fresh, organic fruits and vegetable from around the world most of the year. (Personally, I'm against this luxury. We'll discuss seasonal and local later. For now, it's a gift.)

Growing up, I ate canned fruits except for the grapefruits and oranges my grandparents shipped from Texas, and canned vegetables other than baked potatoes (which do not count as a vegetable in my philosophy). I hated vegetables because I thought they all – even fresh – tasted like canned vegetables.

If you don't always have access to fresh vegetables, frozen green vegetables without the sauce are a healthy option. They are typically flash-frozen right after picking, so they're nutrient dense. Some varieties taste a little too soggy for my preference, yet my husband, who grew up helping his father farm brussels sprouts, swears the frozen ones are the tastiest.

To be clear, when I say eat your vegetables, I am talking about GREEN or water based vegetables such as tomatoes or red and yellow peppers. Choose root vegetables in moderation.

Of course we know veggies are packed with important vitamins and minerals essential for healthy living. Green vegetables are often missing in modern diets. Learning to cook and eat greens may require some experimentation, yet it's essential to good health and looking good. That's because when you nourish yourself with greens, you naturally crowd out the foods that make you gain weight or slow you down.

Green leafy veggies like mixed mesclun greens, spinach, arugula, broccoli, green beans, or asparagus are the most common choices. Less popular, but equally or even more nutrient-dense are kale, brussels sprouts, bok choy, collard greens, watercress, mustard greens, broccoli rabe, endive, radicchio, and napa cabbage. Green cabbage is great raw or in the form of sauerkraut. Spinach, Swiss chard, and beet greens are best eaten in moderation because they are high in oxalic acid, which can deplete calcium from bones and teeth, and, in extreme cases, may lead to osteoporosis.

Nutritionally, greens are high in calcium, magnesium, iron, potassium, phosphorous, zinc, and vitamins A, C, E, and K. They are crammed with fiber, folic acid, chlorophyll, and many other anti-inflammatory micronutrients. I like to pulverize a fresh bunch of parsley and then add it by the quarter-cup to salads, soups, and sauces throughout the week.

Tomatoes, colorful peppers, and mushrooms are all water-based veggies and are smart choices. The rule of thumb is the deeper the rich color, the more nutrient-dense the vegetable. So purple-red beets, orange sweet potatoes, brilliantly-colored varieties of winter squash, and carrots - their deep colors indicate high vitamins and antioxidants.

However, they do have a higher sugar content and hence, higher glycemic index compared to green veggies, so they should be eaten in moderation.

That said, baby carrots as an afternoon snack on the road is a better choice than a granola bar or (heaven forbid) chips or a candy bar. I've heard people say they've cut carrots out of their diet because of sugar, yet they eat tons of candy. Natural sugars found in root vegetables metabolize differently and have natural fiber that slows the sugar absorption which contributes nutritional value. Choosing vegetables wins out.

Now here's your first seemingly contradictory recommendation that I mentioned earlier: learn to drink low-sodium V8. I remember the first time I committed to drinking low-sodium V8 as a low calorie, nutrient-dense snack. I opened the fridge and, seeking willpower, I said out loud, "Come on God, I'm going for the V8!" To this day I still require a bendy straw to suck it down. For me, it was an acquired taste.

What you have in V8 is a lot of vegetables, not necessarily in their most natural state, but, on the go and in a hurry, a V8 fills you up and keeps you from going for something more dangerous. And choose low sodium whenever possible; it's 70% less sodium that regular V8, and most of us get plenty of sodium from the foods we eat, especially when dining out. You'll read more about low-sodium V8 later.

Even when you're trying hard to Be Good, good intentions can go wrong. Use caution when trying to get your fill of vegetables, especially when dining out. Vegetarian dishes in restaurants often contain a lot of butter or cream. Steamed veggies are the wisest choice (but whoa, I really have to be on a mission to order steamed veggies while dining out. Fortunately, whether dining out or cooking at home, you have other options aside from only steamed vegetables.)

One client claimed to only like vegetables with butter. You can alter your tastebuds, weaning yourself off butter (and salt) in stages. Measure a teaspoon of butter, and then use only half. Gradually wean yourself off butter by trying other options. Veggies grilled, roasted or sautéed in olive oil are flavorful choices that don't need butter to be tasty. Flavored vinaigrette dressings can jazz up a plate of veggies. Sometimes I drizzle fresh veggies with vinaigrette dressing before I steam, roast, grill or sauté. When dining out, order any sauce or dressing on the side and drizzle for taste if you must.

When some people hear "leafy green vegetables," they think of iceberg lettuce, but the ordinary, pale lettuce in restaurant salads doesn't have the power-packed goodness of other greens. If it were up to me, iceberg lettuce would be removed from the planet. Even if you love a traditional wedge with blue cheese dressing, popular on many restaurant menus (a splurge only to be eaten occasionally) you could make it using Bibb or romaine for better nutritional value. Get into the habit of adding a variety of dark leafy green vegetables to your daily diet.

Taste preference is entirely up to you but biggest nutritional value is roughly in this order:

Asparagus, watercress, broccoli, brussels sprouts or artichokes are the highest in protein.

Mixed mesclun greens, spinach, arugula, green beans, kale, brussels sprouts, bok choy, collard greens, mustard greens, broccoli rabe, endive, radicchio, spinach, swiss chard, beet greens and napa cabbage are smart choices.

Tomatoes, colorful peppers, and mushrooms count.

Carrots and corn have more sugar than green veggies but are better than processed foods.

What if you could satisfy your sweet tooth with fruits and vegetables?

Fruit contains fiber, vitamins, minerals, and antioxidants that boost the immune system. Low-carb diets often suggest avoiding fruit due to its high sugar content. But in The Marshall Plan, we're not on a diet. We want to eat for a healthy lifestyle. So if you love fresh fruit, especially in season, perhaps at breakfast or occasionally in place of dessert, enjoy it.

In fact, fresh fruit is the wisest choice over other dessert options. Natural sugars found in fresh fruit (as well as root vegetables) metabolize differently and have natural fiber that slows sugar absorption; it contributes nutritional value. There's a difference in how the body metabolizes the natural sugars found in fruit versus white sugar or corn syrup in processed foods (although all excess sugar turns to fat). Even diabetic meal plans allow lower-glycemic-load fruits such as berries, grapefruit, apples, pears, and peaches.

As always, portion size matters, as does frequency and variety. Mix up your choices. You could eat a banana one or two times a week, just don't eat one every day. That's because bananas are relatively high in sugar content, so enjoy one now and then. Be wary of fruit smoothies. They usually contain a banana and, in some chain stores, high sugar/carbohydrate powder added to your drink. Stay away from grocery store yogurt smoothies that contain more sugar and carbohydrates than your desired daily intake.

Based on the "everything in moderation" theory, fruit is a wise choice for breakfast, especially when dining out, over other choices such as sweet breads or buttery eggs and cheese on a muffin. Berries with whole grain cereal or plain yogurt are a delightful treat. Instead of topping your cereal or yogurt with fruit, try the reverse: top a greater portion of fruit with cereal or plain yogurt.

Fruit in the afternoon can be a refreshing snack,

especially on the road when choices are limited. After dinner, a few bites of fruit are a better choice than rich desserts if that satisfies your sweet tooth, especially if you don't trust yourself to have just a bite or two of that high-calorie dessert.

And if you crave something sweet at night, fruit flavored herbal tea is best. If that's not cutting it for you, a handful of fresh blueberries or berries are good. Grapes, although high in natural sugar, are better than candy or manufactured snacks. And Special K cereal with chocolate bits is not an option, despite what the commercial says.

Sugar content in fresh fruit varies as does portion size, but an overall guideline (and it varies from chart to chart) of smart choices based on glycemic load is: Avocados, all berries, melons, grapefruit, plum kiwi, peaches, pear, grapes, oranges, apples, mango, papaya. bananas, to name a few.

Let's close this chapter on fruits and vegetables with a quick discussion of juices and juicing.

As you've read, fresh fruit and vegetables are the wisest choice. The same holds true for fresh juices: fresh-squeezed orange and grapefruit are good, but store-bought juices are typically bad because they often contain more sugar. Store-bought lemonade can have as much sugar as a can of cola.

Similarly, homemade smoothies are better for you because you can control the ingredients (fresh or frozen fruit, skim or low fat milk or just ice) whereas, as I mentioned earlier, store-bought smoothies typically contain a lot of sugar. Read the labels, especially on the ones you think are the healthiest. Some are two servings per container and up to 40+ grams of sugar in one of those servings.

"Juicing" is a popular craze and it's good for you. Who would ever guess kale and celery could taste so good when you add a cucumber, a little lemon, and green apples. And ginger is a great anti-inflammatory agent, if you like the flavor.

Juicing is a lot of work, getting the flavors just right isn't easy, and frankly, cleanup can be a nightmare. If you're up for a green veggie juice, try one from an expert. It's a great filling snack or meal replacement if you're so inclined, and it's packed with nutrients you need when you're on the quest for optimal health. Yes, buying from an expert can be pricey, but as my father would say, it's big bang for your buck.

The foundation of this program is simple: fill up on fresh fruits and vegetables, primarily green food. Whenever possible, choose organic. But eating non-organic greens is much better than not eating any greens at all!

When you look at your plate, one half to two-thirds should be vegetables. Consider green food as "freebies" – you can eat as much as you want. And there are so many greens to choose from. Find greens that you love and eat them often. When you get bored with your favorites, be adventurous and try greens you've never heard of. When you go to a farmer's market, you'll see what's in season. Ask the vendor how they would prepare them. Most likely you can steam, sauté, roast or grill them with a sprinkle of olive oil and a few seasonings. It's crazy easy to figure out how to prepare just about anything these days. When in doubt just Google "easy recipes for …"

Quick take-away:
Green Veggies are your best friend. Fill up on greens at every meal and for every snack whenever possible.

CHAPTER 5

Good Carbs, Bad Carbs

IT IS ESSENTIAL to learn to differentiate between good, healthy, whole-grain carbohydrates, also known as complex carbs, and bad, white, processed carbohydrates.

In theory, each meal should contain a ratio of 40% carbohydrates, 30% protein, and 30% good fats. Barry Sears calls this the Zone Diet. But we're not following a diet. You want to learn the difference between good carbs and bad carbs so you can make smart choices day in and day out so you eat a balanced diet.

The most important element to emphasize is that FRUITS AND VEGETABLES are CARBOHYDRATES. So if you eat 50% fruits and vegetables at each meal, you're getting most of your carbohydrates from low-calorie, low-fat, nutrient-dense foods. (You may add healthy fats (olive oil) to the preparation of your vegetables so they're more satisfying. We'll delve into deeper detail about healthy fats and lean protein in a later chapter.)

Most people hear the word "carbohydrate" and think

bread, pasta, and rice, and that's true. It's important to know the difference: good carbs are whole-grain, unprocessed, unrefined, and close to their naturally grown state; bad carbs are refined, processed, bleached white flour carbohydrates.

Bad carbs metabolize into sugar which stores as fat in your body. You don't need white carbs for energy even if you're training for a marathon. You get the biggest bang for your buck when you choose whole grains, but you must do so wisely.

Because of the popularity of whole grains, food labels can be misleading. Unfortunately, FDA regulations aren't strict enough to prevent food manufacturers from distorting the truth. Packaged breads and cereals are the worst offenders. Many "whole grain" cereals are loaded with sugar, and some breads labelled "natural" or "whole wheat" are still made with bleached flour. Most breakfast cereals tout whole grain on the labels but often contain hidden sugars and excess carbs. Granola is often high in fat and sugar.

Steel cut oats, a slow-cooking oatmeal, is better than instant oatmeal because it's closer to the natural form. Instant oatmeal has a higher glycemic index than slow-cooking oatmeal. A higher glycemic index means the carbs are absorbed more quickly, causing your blood sugar to rise faster, which means you metabolize them faster, and excess sugar turns to fat. Furthermore, artificially flavored oatmeal contains more sugar.

In a pinch, plain instant oatmeal is acceptable. To add flavor to either plain instant oatmeal or steel-cut oats, you can add natural sugars like raw honey, agave nectar, fresh fruits, antioxidant-rich cinnamon, nuts, or even a smidge of almond butter for protein and omegas. It's important to know the difference so you can make educated choices.

Good carbs, also known as complex carbs and whole grains, are a good source of vitamins as well as fiber, which helps keep digestion and cholesterol in check. Whole grains like bulgar wheat, barley, quinoa, kamut, or spelt (to name a few of the many available), as well as whole grain breads, pastas, and brown rice are good choices in moderation. Less than one half cup per meal is a generous serving. Personally, I try to keep it to less than half cup one time a day. When you're just getting started, two quarter to half cup servings of complex carbs is acceptable.

If you love sushi, experiment with brown rice sushi, and pull off as much rice as you possibly can. (I've pulled off at least half cup of rice while still eating about a quarter of a cup of rice with the sushi.) These hidden calories sabotage your goals. Ordering sashimi helps balance out the carb load.

If you love pasta with red tomato sauce, try a quarter cup of sauce drizzled over half a cup of whole grain pasta such as whole wheat, kamut, or brown rice pasta. Yes, some of these options require time to alter your tastebuds. If you're a purist and you want white flour pasta bolognese, you can have it on occasion as a splurge once you've met your goals.

Try to eat whole grain carbs earlier in the day versus at your evening meal so you can expend the energy. A balanced meal of protein and whole grains will sustain your energy levels throughout the day.

Remember, this is not a life sentence. You don't have to deprive yourself forever. You just want to Be Good most of the time, and make a cognitive choice to Be Bad.

All types of potatoes are starchy carbohydrates, and starchy carbs metabolize similarly to white carbs. As with everything, there are smarter choices, and of course how they're prepared matters.

Sweet potatoes have more nutrients than white potatoes. Try them baked whole and limit your add-ons to herbs and just a little salt and pepper. Sliced and roasted preparation allows you portion control. Mashed sweet potatoes makes a yummy comfort food delicious enough to serve at Thanksgiving.

As for white potatoes, red new and fingerling potatoes, baked, roasted, or boiled are good choices as you can limit your portion size. Leave the skins on as they contain more nutrients. Baked large white potatoes, stuffed or double stuffed are not your friend. Sliced and roasted potatoes aren't the worst things for you, but not the best choices if you're trying to Be Good.

Throughout these chapters you'll learn smart choices for other add-ons for baked and roasted potatoes. Butter, sour cream, and marshmallow fluff (think Thanksgiving casseroles) are not acceptable.

Mashed or whipped potatoes are extremely dangerous when dining out as they are typically loaded with butter, heavy cream, or milk. If you really LOVE them and have to have them, make them at home using vegetable or chicken stock with salt and pepper. If you have to use milk, cut it with the veggie or chicken stock. Of course, choosing mashed potatoes or french fries intentionally to Be Bad, is an occasional treat, depending on your goals.

Mashed sweet potato, made healthier at home, is a more nutrient-dense option. Or if you're Being Good, try cauliflower mash using cauliflower in place of potatoes - it's an acquired taste for some, yet it's a good way to get your veggies in while you're Being Good.

Beans and legumes are some of the best sources of protein and fiber, yet are often omitted from meal plans. If you're not likely to eat them as a main meal, try adding a quarter cup of garbanzo, black beans, white kidney beans, or lentils to a salad, and look for recipes for legume based side dishes. You'll be pleasantly surprised.

If you're a newcomer to beans and legumes, don't be distressed by preparation instructions requiring overnight soaking. Many types are easily accessible canned, packed in water (low sodium options are best).

If you've never really tried legumes, experiment with small portions at Whole Foods or Fresh Market, where they offer pre-made salads and sides. Hummus is a yummy dip made primarily of mashed garbanzo beans, olive oil, and tahini.

Remember, too much of even a good thing can sabotage your goals. Legumes are calorie-dense, so be mindful of your portions. And be wary of Mexican-style beans cooked in lard. LARD - just typing the word makes me shiver!

Carbohydrates get a bad rap because anything over-consumed or not nutritionally digestible becomes fat. Sugar has no food value and metabolizes to fat; flours, including whole wheat, metabolize similarly to sugar (two slices of wheat toast metabolizes like two tablespoons of white sugar). You get the drift. That's why even when eating whole grains, portion control is important. A quarter to a half cup maximum, a few times per week, is Being Good.

Carbs are preferred in this order:
1. Green veggies
2. Fresh fruit
3. Root vegetables: carrots, beets, sweet potatoes, new potatoes
4. Squash
5. Raw nuts - good protein, but high fat. It's "good fat," but fat is still fat
6. Legumes - good proteins, calorie dense
7. Whole grains: quinoa, barley, kamut, spelt, brown rice to name a few
8. White potatoes, rice, or pasta
9. Breads: whole grain versus white
10. Cereals: steel cut oats are the safest; look for added sugar in packaged cereals and oatmeal
11. Frozen yogurt or ice cream
12. Baked sweets: pastry, cookies, cakes, pies
13. Candy

You've most likely heard about the gluten-free fad. Yes, for many people it's important to watch gluten intake as it contributes to many food allergies that can be difficult to detect. If you fear you might be allergic to gluten, you should see a Health Counselor, nutritionist, or doctor who can guide you through a series of tests to determine if gluten-free will ease your symptoms.

If you choose to reduce gluten in your diet that's easier, yet you still need to know a lot about food content. In The Marshall Plan, it is easy to reduce gluten during the Being Good phase and allow yourself some freedom and flexibility on a Being Bad day.

Hopefully you're also aware that bad carbs and sugar contribute to diabetes. Pre-diabetes is on an epidemic rise in people between the ages of 15 – 60. Sixty use to be the norm for detecting Type II Diabetes.

Carbohydrates that digest slowly into your bloodstream will help reduce gluten allergy symptoms and help prevent pre-diabetes. These are foods like sweet potatoes, cooked carrots (either steamed or lightly sautéed), quinoa, brown rice, lentils, chickpeas, black beans, and fruits such as apples or peaches. These are all considered low glycemic load. Check out the many lists of glycemic index and glycemic load for your favorite foods and see where you might want to make some changes.

As the popularity of "no carb" diets fizzles, choices are less about rigid rules and more about enjoying everything in moderation. Portion control matters, as does the need to read your labels and seek fresh whole ingredients.

Quick take-away: Veggies are good carbs – kinda like a freebie. Complex carbs or whole grains are good in moderation. Don't be fooled by labels.

CHAPTER 6

Lean Protein

LEAN PROTEIN IS a key ingredient when trying to lose or maintain your weight because eating the right amount of protein can help you build muscle, which increases your metabolism.

The word LEAN should come as no surprise to you. Lean protein is low in saturated fat; saturated fat causes obesity and heart disease. And, as with everything else we've discussed, you should look for lean protein, whether vegetable or animal, as close to its natural form and ideally organic. Humane treatment of animal processing is a hot topic, but for the purposes of The Marshall Plan, if you like to eat meat, poultry, or seafood, enjoy.

Avocados, a fruit, are a good source of heart healthy protein, yet they're calorie-dense; vegetables like asparagus, broccoli, brussels sprouts, artichoke, watercress and cauliflower are low-calorie yet provide some protein. You can get good protein from nuts, legumes, and tofu (versus genetically modified soy products,) but again, mind your portion control as they are more calorie dense.

Lean protein can also include certain cuts of red meat, pork, and turkey or chicken breast meat (versus darker meat or duck). Eggs are a good source of protein in moderation as they are high in cholesterol. Seafood is a great source of protein, although many species are endangered or are contaminated with mercury, which is why everything in moderation is important.

Protein is found in dairy, such as milk or cheese, yet these choices are high in saturated fat. Low-fat varieties of dairy are better than non-fat varieties as non-fat dairy products are metabolized quickly as carbohydrates. Note too, that they are moving away from the fresh food guideline because they're more processed.

When choosing lean protein, the choice is entirely up to you and your preferences. Whichever protein you choose, preparation is key to maintain the healthy element of your choice. Adding flavor really matters because you want to eat satisfying, good food.

Ideally, add flavor using fresh organic spices. Dried organic spices in your cabinet are handy to have on hand. Clean out your current stash and replenish with a variety of new flavors. Simply Organic has a sixteen-count spice rack for about $55 which will add zest to your home cooking.

There are a number of healthy, flavored marinades for meat, poultry, and seafood. Look for vinaigrette-based dressings, low sodium/low sugar sauces or marinades, and use them in moderation.

Baking is a great, clean option as is grilling over a

non-charcoal grill. Charcoal grilling is okay as long you are mindful about carcinogens from charring meat or too much smoke.

Sautéing, or lightly pan frying is flavorful, but again you must be mindful of the amount of oil you use. Olive oil is the healthiest choice of all the oils, but keep in mind even with olive oil, fat is fat.

In most cases of meat, be it pork or steak, trimming the fat is essential to a healthy cut as well as portion size. Three to four ounces is about the diameter of your palm.

Nuts and legumes are good sources of vegetarian protein, but they're calorie-dense, so be mindful of your portions as well as preparation. Raw nuts are best, roasted unsalted are okay. Eat nuts slowly, one at a time, as a healthy portion size is just seven to 10 nuts. If you're tossing back a handful or two, you're consuming way too many calories.

Nut butters are a popular source of protein. When buying either peanut butter or almond butter, you want to be sure you are getting the most natural form. The ingredient list should only include the nut (almond or peanut) and maybe some salt. There should not be any added oils or other fillers. The nutrition facts for peanut and almond butter are about the same amount of calories and fat. The micronutrients in almond butter provides beneficial vitamins and antioxidants that aid in body function and prevent disease. But if you like the flavor of cashew or peanut butter, choose that option now and again. It's okay to mix it up.

41

If you're exercising, you may be hungrier overall, and protein will help you feel more full.

But, as in anything, too much of a good thing will add pounds, so you need to know how much you're consuming. Typically, you require half a gram of protein per pound of your weight. So divide your weight by two, and that's approximately the number of grams you require per day. For most people that comes to about 20-30 grams of protein at each meal. Extremely high-protein diets can cause stiff joints, constipation, and can be taxing on your liver. As with everything, mindful, moderate consumption is key.

Try to eat your largest meal at lunch if possible. Three to four ounces of lean protein with two sides of vegetables should do the trick during the Being Good phase at home. Diversity matters. Experiment with a variety of cuts of meat or poultry, or types of fish, and a variety of preparation. And even in a restaurant, order your lean protein with vegetables and hold the rice or mashed potatoes.

The same portion size holds true for poultry, and white meat is more lean than dark meat. With ground meat, turkey, or chicken it can be tricky to know what the restaurant may have added – eggs, dairy, or breadcrumbs can't easily be detected.

Seafood is typically a healthy option as long as it's not fried and smothered in sauce. (Remember to order sauce on the side or, if it comes floating in sauce, move the piece to a smaller plate.)

Depending on your preference, there are several

choices of lean protein. Some more common good choices are:

- Avocado or veggies like asparagus, watercress, broccoli, or brussels sprouts.

- Seafood, white meat poultry, lean cuts of pork, or steak like filet mignon.

- Dry cheeses like parmesan, feta, ricotta have some protein.

- Almonds, walnuts, cashews, brazil nuts, hazelnuts raw or in nut butters are good protein, but not so lean.

Quick take-away: Choose lean protein to stave off hunger, with LEAN being the operative word!

CHAPTER 7

Dairy: You Decide.

DAIRY IS A controversial topic.

In general, dairy is perceived as not good for you. Most dairy is processed, so you're not consuming dairy in its most natural form. For many, dairy is a main cause of food allergies. For others, dairy slows down weight loss because it's loaded with saturated fats and high in cholesterol.

As for butter – you really want to minimize your intake. On bread? Hardly ever. Bread should be so delicious it doesn't need butter, otherwise, just say no. In cooking, olive oil is a more heart-healthy choice than butter, but baking is the best reason to just go for the real thing. Skip manmade concoctions like margarine or butter substitutes.

Restaurant kitchens often use some form of fat-laden dairy as filler or thickening agent in many dishes. You'll want to stay away from cream-based salad dressings and soups, especially those with the word "bisque" in the title. Always ask your server if cream has been added to a soup and, when in doubt, just say no.

Typically, salad dressings with the word "vinaigrette" in their name are oil based, not cream based. Caesar salad is not a healthy choice. In fact, Caesar salad dressing is one of the most saturated fat-laden dressings available, and because of how it's made it doesn't serve well on the side. If you love it, choose knowingly. If you're at a place where healthy choices are extremely limited and Caesar salad looks like the best option (at least it's romaine lettuce vs. evil iceberg) ask for no dressing, and use squeezes of fresh lemon juice instead. You might even learn to like it that way.

Yogurt is another choice often perceived as healthy. Many people reach for a fruit yogurt for a quick lunch or snack on the go and think they're making a healthy choice. Unfortunately, the ones that taste good usually have lots of added sugar. Plain fresh yogurt is good for you, but it may contain more saturated fat than you need.

When choosing packaged yogurts, plain Greek-style yogurt is a good choice to cook with or eat on its own. You can add extras such as fresh fruit, antioxidant-rich cinnamon and/or raw honey or agave nectar if you must. If you're buying packaged yogurt with fruit, look for low fat and check the label for sugar content. Anything higher than 14 to16 grams of sugar per serving is high, and you'll be surprised by how many brands and flavors are in that range.

Low- or non-fat options are suggested in moderation because when manufacturers take out fat, they tend to add sugar to enhance flavor, especially in yogurts and ice cream. Sugar adds bad carbohydrates that turn to fat. Even all-natural, low-fat brands often have added sugar to compensate for less fat. That being said, frozen yogurt is a better option than ice cream on a frequent basis, so depending on how good you want to be, some of the new, more natural varieties of frozen yogurt is a reasonable *treat*. The key is frequency; rather than having yogurt three or four times a week, can you Be Good, enjoying one serving just once or twice a month?

Soy, almond, or rice milk are popular non-dairy choices, but again they can be loaded with sugar. One percent milk is a better choice than those alternatives if you have to have milk in your diet.

Non-fat dairy such as skim milk, cottage cheese, sour cream, or yogurt metabolize as a carbohydrate, not a protein as is the common perception.

Cheese, ahh, glorious cheese. The good news is cheese has a low glycemic index; the bad news is cheddar, Swiss, Colby, and American cheese are all bad fat culprits, high in cholesterol, and play havoc on your waistline.

Treat cheese like chocolate: choose to consume cheese as a treat, savoring every bite. If your sandwich comes with a choice of cheese, just say, "No cheese, please" if you're trying to Be Good. Shredded cheese in your salad? Pull some off to the side. French onion soup with melted cheese on top, do I need to say it? Just say no.

Better cheese choices are parmesan, mozzarella, feta, ricotta, and goat cheese when being moderately good.

Low-fat versions of cream cheese, sour cream, and

mayonnaise are occasionally acceptable, typically in recipe replacement and in moderation of course.

Indulge in really good cheese as a treat when you are intentionally Being Bad.

Minimize dairy consumption by never eating dairy at home, only in restaurants, especially since you can't control most of the ingredients when dining out. Personally, I love a good cheese plate; I never have cheese at home and enjoy it at a restaurant once in a while. This cognitive effort helps keep my dairy consumption in moderation. You don't want to deprive yourself of things you love because, in the long run you'll crave them and overindulge.

Remember, we're trying to eat mainly whole foods, in their most fresh natural state, so processed dairy is a questionable choice. In the world of Being Good to Be Bad, dairy leans to the Bad side: it's fine in moderation, as a special treat once you've met your goals.

The Marshall Plan promotes balanced, smart lifestyle choices. That might mean cooking with dairy products in moderation, using ingredients that lean toward the light side. Good fats versus bad fats play an important role when selecting dairy products for at home consumption.

As in every category, it's important to remember that diversity matters and moderation is key.

Quick take-away: Keep dairy limited. Choose wisely.

CHAPTER 8

Good Fats versus Bad Fats

YOU DON'T HAVE to be a nutrition expert to sort out the difference between good fats and bad fats, and it's important to know which are which.

Good fats are vital to healthy digestion, increased energy, and decreased body fat through a more active metabolism, glowing skin, hair, and nails, and elevated mood through brain activity. Good fats are essential in vitamin D absorption, and they boost your immune system. Some studies even suggest that depression increased during the low fat/no fat diet craze in the 80s and 90s.

The goal is to understand the difference between good, healthy fats and bad, unhealthy fats so you can moderate your intake of good fat and decrease saturated and trans fat in your eating strategy.

Good fats, also known as monounsaturated fats, are highest in olive, sesame, or canola oils, nuts, and soybeans, and are the most heart-healthy fats. Besides protecting your heart, decreasing your risk for certain cancer, and helping you maintain a healthy weight, sources of monounsaturated fats add flavor to your lean protein and vegetables, and can easily can be flavored with herbs, chillies, or garlic.

One of the more astounding facts about switching to monounsaturated fats from trans fats and saturated fats is that you'll lose weight and belly fat. Hello, good fat reduces belly fat! (And you'll recall that excess carbs and sugar turns to belly fat, so you're winning a battle by eating good fat.)

Polyunsaturated fats are more complicated. The polyunsaturated fats found in avocados, lean poultry, and fish are good for you, especially the Omega-3 fats found in fish such as salmon. Fish oil or Omega-3 supplements are recommended to ensure you're getting enough Omega-3 fats in your diet.

On the other hand, polyunsaturated oils such as sunflower, safflower, or soybean oil are less desirable because of their molecular make-up. It starts to get confusing as charts vary and it's difficult to monitor, especially while dining out. For simplicity's sake, stay away from saturated fats, choose optimal heart-healthy monounsaturated fats when cooking at home, and don't sweat the details about polyunsaturated fats when you're dining out for a good time. You know if you're ordering grilled or sautéed chicken breast or seafood at a better restaurant, it's a smarter choice.

Saturated fats and trans fats – the really bad fats – are bad for your waistline and your overall health, but the problem is that they typically taste really good.

You most likely know that bad fats cause obesity and heart disease. Saturated fats are high in cholesterol.

Trans fats hit the media in 2006 when new food label laws required trans fats to be listed on all labels. What's deceiving is many labels claim to have "no trans fat," yet still contain saturated fat.

I have a friend who sends an email to help her children sell Girl Scout cookies. She always notes, "No trans fat." But those cookies still have bad, saturated fat that sabotages your healthy weight goals, in addition to sugar and empty calories. So don't be fooled by labels that tout "no trans fats." Look for the amount of *saturated* fat on the label.

Also be wary of marketing claims that mayonnaise made with olive oil is a healthy choice. They may have some olive oil, but not olive oil in its purist form, as The Marshall Plan philosophy recommends. Some brands contain saturated fats, some don't. You have to read your labels carefully.

I often substitute a combination of plain yogurt and dijon mustard in place of low-fat mayonnaise or sour cream. Play with it to find the flavors you like best. The Marshall Plan is all about eating what you love in moderation, and it's your choice how Good you want to be, and how seriously you want to see results.

I personally have always detested the taste and abhor the sight of mayonnaise. It most likely goes back to my no-fat diet days, where all I envision is globules of fat, and truthfully, mayonnaise is just that. So if you really want to Be Good, just say no to mayonnaise.

Butter and margarine are another source of bad fat. In the late 1950s and 60s, margarine was touted as the heart-healthy, low-cholesterol alternative to artery clogging butter. You know that adage, what sounds too good to be true isn't? Same holds true with margarine and other butter substitutes. The trans fats found in stick versions of margarine negate any over-marketed benefits. Soft-spread margarine does have less trans fat, but it's still not all it's cracked up to be.

Remember the premise of The Marshall Plan: eat whole foods in the form closest to natural. If you want to bake or cook with butter, use real butter. And – you guessed it – be intentional and use it in moderation. If you're making grandma's favorite cookie recipe, use the butter and enjoy the cookies – just not every day.

Whatever choices you make, keep in mind that fat is fat. You can gain weight from too much good fat, so monitor your intake carefully. Yes, a handful of raw almonds are 15 grams of good fat, rich in fiber, protein, antioxidants, and allover good for you, but several handfuls a day are too many fat grams – good or bad.

The simple approach: learn to love the foods that are commonly known to have good fats and stay away from bad fats as much as possible except when you choose to Be Bad.

Convenience food technology brings us the joy of fat free Twinkies, cookies, candies, ice cream, cream cheese, sour cream, and yogurt, to name a few normally high-fat foods people did not want to go without. And believe me - guilty as charged. I was in heaven devouring a box of fat free cookies. Yes, a *box*, not knowing that to create yummy flavor without fat, manufacturers increase sugar and other manmade flavor additives. That box of cookies (and other fat-free products) is poison and no help for your waistline.

The theory is, if you really want a Twinkie or a box of Oreos, just go for it. Unless, of course, you're on The Marshall Plan and you know better. Wouldn't you prefer a fresh-baked cookie rather than one from a box, if you were really going to Be Bad, after Being so Good to meet your goals?

Some high protein diets disregard the difference between good and bad fats, and are only successful when you strictly follow the plan to get the chemical reaction that results in rapid weight loss. This method can be successful for extremely obese people who need to jumpstart their weight-loss journey. But the original strategy behind this method has been distorted. In order to create the chemical reaction that induces weight loss, you had to follow strict rules. I recall being at a party with a friend who was chowing down on slices of American cheese because it was protein, while also eating potato chips and cake. It was a very self-destructive distortion of the high fat diet.

Diets *shouldn't* last long. Eventually, we all have to learn to eat healthy and balanced meals in order to look good and feel good. The Marshall Plan promotes healthy lifestyle choices. Good fats can help you metabolize your food better so you look good and feel good. Remember: fat is still fat, good or bad, so be aware of moderate portion size.

The skinny on fats:

- When dining out, don't sweat the details of polyunsaturated fats.
- Stay away from saturated fats found in lard, butter, and all kinds of yummy foods.
- Trans fat are a man-made nightmare, but beware trans-fat-free labels.
- Choose olive or sesame oils to cook with at home.

Quick take-away:
Know and eat good fats in moderation. Choose bad fats intentionally, to Be Bad.

CHAPTER 9

Sugar

HIDDEN SUGARS, ESPECIALLY in so-called "healthy" foods, can really sabotage your best efforts to eat healthy while trying to lose or maintain weight. Excess sugar turns to fat – period, end. The fat-free trend in the 90's failed us because manufacturers added sugar to compensate for the loss of flavor caused by taking out the fat.

There's nothing wrong with consuming a little sugar; it's just that we tend consume too much, and it matters whether it's natural or processed. Some of my clients stay away from fruit because of the sugar content, yet still consume candy. Well, it's your choice, but, if approximately 40 grams of sugar per day is acceptable, it would seem that your best choice is to get those 40 grams from natural, nutrient-dense fruits and vegetables.

Naturally-occurring sugars are those which are an inherent part of a food or drink, which explains why some foods just naturally taste sweeter than others. Many fruits have more naturally-occurring sugars than veggies do, causing the fruit to taste sweeter. You should never need to add sweeteners to seasonally fresh fruit.

(Remember, you can train your tastebuds and reduce your desire for super-sweet foods.)

Consuming sugar in moderation is key, as is knowing processed sugars from natural. If you're watching glycemic load, you should know that natural sugars are thought not to cause as quick a spike in blood sugar (since they help the body absorb sugar) in the ways refined and processed sugars can. Of course, any amount of sugar can cause blood sugar to climb.

Natural sugars found in fruits and vegetables are better for you, but remember that even natural sugar is a sugar. If you're a normally healthy person, it's okay to eat higher-sugar-content fruits and starchy vegetables occasionally, just not daily. If you diversify and mind your portion sizes, you can eat almost any fruit you want.

However, note that bananas, carrots, and potatoes are known as high-sugar fruit and vegetables, and so they have a high glycemic index. This matters if you have a family history of Type II diabetes or if you've been told you're Pre-Type II Diabetes. In this case, you need to become familiar with foods with high glycemic index or glycemic load so you can minimize your intake. Check out the on-line lists of fruit and their glycemic load. You'll see that the lists vary, but in general the differences are minimal.

When consuming manufactured foods (versus whole food fruit or root vegetables), a sugar content of between 15 and 18 grams is acceptable. Read the labels! To really manage your sugar intake, you need to a be a sugar super-sleuth. You might be surprised to learn that some manufactured tomato soup contains 14 grams of sugar per cup - you'd think a veggie soup would be a freebie, but it's not so. Being a super sugar sleuth, I found a boxed, low sodium tomato soup with only 2 grams of sugar so you have read your labels.

Most packaged juices or smoothies are ladened with sugar. Fruited yogurts tend to average 24 grams or higher, and should be consumed in moderation (as in once a week, or twice month if you're serious about cutting sugar.) Instead of the fruited yogurt, treat yourself to a plain Greek yogurt and add raw honey and your own fresh fruit. Better yet, top your fresh fruit with a dollop of Greek yogurt.

Breakfast cereals are another sneaky, waistline-sabotaging culprit. The food industry is under tons of scrutiny for misleading labels touting natural and whole grain. Until that's resolved, you need to know how to read labels if you want to identify the healthiest choices. Most breakfast cereals contain a lot of sugar additives as well as other preservatives. Even supposed whole-grain cereals, granola, or fiber bars include excess sugars that sabotage your waistline.

And, of course, portion size matters. When you read the content label, note the portion size. Take out your measuring cup and pour out a serving. Put it in your bowl and take a look at the measured portion size. Then make a note to yourself: do not eat more than this, and only a few times a week.

Other sugar-concealing culprits? Many processed condiments such as ketchup, BBQ sauce, some tomato sauce, honey mustard, teriyaki, and some cocktail sauces have a high sugar content, as do maple syrup, honey, jellies and jams. Choose light or sugar-free versions occasionally.

Remember though, when a food is promoted as "light" some other ingredient is often added to compensate for flavor. For example, light sugar might have more fat, while non-fat products such as yogurt, ice cream, or cheese, will have more sugar.

The type of sugar matters. Anything in its natural form is a better choice. Raw sugar is better than white sugar. When reading labels, look for natural sweeteners: raw honey is packed with antioxidants, making it a smart choice in moderation. Agave nectar is a natural substitute as a topping or in baking, but it is still a syrup processed from the agave plant, so use it in moderation. Stevia, another plant derivative, is good in small quantities for coffee or tea drinkers.

Stay away from anything with added sugar content that ends is "ose" such as sucrose, glucose, fructose, and even lactose in milk and dairy products, as well as manufactured sweeteners such as saccharin and aspartame. The manufacturers of high-fructose corn syrup are trying to fool you into believing that it's a natural derivative of corn. In fact, they've recently tried to rename high fructose corn syrup as "corn sugar" to camouflage the bad associations with obesity and diabetes.

Do I need to waste anyone's time discussing soda?

Drinking soda is out of the question. With 39 grams of sugar and no nutritional value, why would you waste empty calories and blow your daily allotment of sugar?

You're better off enjoying a scoop of ice cream or some other outrageous dessert on occasion, savoring every morsel. Even diet soda with artificial sweeteners can sabotage your efforts to get off sugar. Consumed on a regular basis, artificial sweeteners actually increase your cravings for sweets.

As I've said before and will keep on saying, the secret to success is to seek whole foods in their natural state. When you need fast food – which means manufactured food that comes in a box or container, *read your labels.* And remember, everything in moderation; not every day.

I'm never one to say deprive yourself of all things sugar – after all, the main philosophy behind The Marshall Plan is to eat, drink and look good. Just choose your sugars wisely and be aware of hidden sugars, especially in so-called healthy foods.

The sweet summary about sugar:
–   Natural sugars found in fruits are good for an average healthy person.
–   Natural sugars found in raw honey, agave nectar and raw maple sugar has more antioxidants but are still metabolized as a sugar.
–   Processed sugar one minute on the lips, goes right to the hips - proceed with caution!

Quick take-away: Know the difference between natural sugar and processed sugar. Be a super-sleuth for hidden sugar in processed food.

CHAPTER 10

Water

You ALWAYS HEAR that drinking eight to 10 glasses of water a day is a secret to weight loss. Well, you don't necessarily have to drink eight to 10 glasses each day, but you can never drink enough water, so just keep drinking as much as you can all day long. Eight, eight-ounce glasses is a good goal, but it's not always convenient. Don't wait until you're thirsty and on the way to dehydration. Listen to your body. Sip water throughout the day. There are free apps for counting glasses of water; it's fun to monitor your intake for a few weeks to learn whether you need to bump it up a bit. Water, which is processed through your kidneys, is a great way to flush toxins out of your system.

In many communities, tap water is not safe to drink and bottled water isn't necessarily better. The ideal option is to filter your own water with a reverse osmosis filter on your kitchen tap, or use a pitcher with a carbon filter. Drinking from a glass or stainless steel bottle is the most environmentally friendly method.

Naturally, the warmer the weather, the more water

you need. If you work out heavily on extremely hot days, you might want to consider electrolyte-enhanced water. Depending on the intensity of your workout, eight to 10 ounces of an electrolyte-enhanced water every day or every other day is good, but you don't have to drink these amped-up waters all day. Be mindful of caloric drinks if weight loss is one of your goals. The low calorie options are not close to a natural state, so choose wisely.

Excessive amounts of plain water in extreme heat can actually flush out your electrolytes. This happened to a friend at an outdoor ropes course in Austin, Texas, in mid-July. As the conference leader instructed, she drank tons of water while sweating profusely in 115* heat during the activities. That evening she felt nauseous and dizzy and was taken to the hospital where they replenished her system with a vitamin-nourished IV. It was like an extreme hangover, the same symptoms of dehydration. Extreme heat is definitely a reason to supplement your water intake with electrolyte enhanced beverages. Read the labels for low sugar and the least amount of man-made chemicals. Electrolyte enhanced waters should be the exception, not the norm.

Smart choices tell you to choose water over diet soda (I know you'd never choose regular soda.) In summer, when it's really hot and I consume more water than normal, sometimes I crave something else, a little sweet, around midday. Once a week or so, I might have a diet soda or Crystal Light raspberry tea or lemonade (I love an occasional vodka & Crystal Light lemonade in summer.) The key is to only drink artificially sweetened beverages on occasion: some nutritionists say that satiating that sweet tooth with artificial sweeteners actually encourages cravings. By avoiding artificial sweeteners you can train your brain to give up its desire for sugar. A better option would be to make iced tea using herbal fruit flavored teas, adding raw honey or agave nectar if need be.

Quick take-away:
It's best to sip water all day long. Start with a big glass first thing in the morning and keep drinking all day long. Be mindful of water consumption after 8pm, otherwise eliminating all that water might keep you up during the night.

CHAPTER 11

Clear Liquids

UP UNTIL A certain point in the aging process, it seems like calories from alcohol don't matter. Then one day you wake up and bam, you're exercising, eating, and drinking as usual yet you're up a few pounds and they won't come off.

Alcohol turns to sugar, sugar turns to fat, and your pants are too tight. For party people, and you know who you are, it's time to be aware of calories in alcohol. (The original title of this book was *The Marshall Plan – The Party Girl's Guide to Eat, Drink & be Merry*.)

In the 1980s, I drank vodka and club soda with a twist as my "diet" cocktail. In the 1990s, *Sex and the City* created a cultural shift, re-introducing cosmopolitans and other fruity, tasty martinis into our mainstream party menu. In 1997, I drank my first mojito at La Bodeguita del Medio, Ernest Hemingway's bar in Havana. Although I served cocktails throughout the 1980's to mid 90's, I had never heard of a mojito. Yet within a few years the mint-mashing, time-consuming mixologist trend had taken restaurants and nightclubs across the world by storm.

The reason those tasty concoctions go down so easy is added sugar. Same with Margaritas: if they're made with a sour mix, you're consuming high sugar and sodium.

Margaritas, mojitos, and fancy martinis can run to 250–300 calories per cocktail. Yikes! Have two, and that's nearly half your daily caloric allotment. If you're making them at home try stevia, the all-natural sugar substitute, or Skinny Girl's mix: it's *not good* for you, just not as bad. I'm skeptical of ordering skinny cocktails in a restaurant because you never know if you're really getting one. I only order one while sitting at the bar where I can watch the bartender make it for me - and that's once in a blue moon.

Drinking clear liquids is the key to success. Light beer, white wine, champagne, or vodka or gin with club soda (or better, sparkling or seltzer water since they contain no salt) and a squeeze of lemon, lime, or orange can be quite refreshing. Rum, tequila and whiskey do not have any more sugar than clear liquids, but can have higher calorie content and are often combined with sugary mixers. Stay away from liqueurs that do have higher sugar content. Think clear liquids, it's an easy rule of thumb to remember.

Alcohol consumption is a frequent topic in social circles and current research as well. Is a glass of wine a night too much? Studies show a glass of wine per night is healthier than consuming nothing during the week, and then seven to eight drinks per weekend. But truthfully, do we ever consume just one? Dry nights during the week (you decide how many are right for you) are a good idea if you know you consume more drinks on the weekend, and/or are trying to cut calories to watch your waistline. On the other hand, if moderation is your thing, enjoy your drink or two whenever.

Clear liquids like light beer, champagne, white wine, vodka or gin with sparkling water or club soda if you're in a bar are your best options for a libation.

Quick take-away:
Look for no sugar, no simple syrup options, only drinking clear liquids when enjoying a libation or two, or three...

CHAPTER 12

Stock the Fridge

THE BEST WAY to avoid overeating is to simply not have a lot of food around. Try to keep your refrigerator and cupboard contents to a minimum and, as we've already discussed, the fewer packaged foods the better.

That being said, it's good to have healthy choices readily available at home so you can make smart decisions when you're hungry. The list below will give you an idea of what's good to have on hand. Fresh is always ideal, but I include some packaged goods for emergencies and for when you're in a rush.

Look for low sugar, low fat, low sodium options, remembering to also check for added ingredients that you *don't* want.

- Fresh or Frozen Fruits & Veggies (frozen in bags are the easiest and most handy)
- Strawberries
- Raspberries
- Blackberries
- Blueberries
- Cantaloupe or honeydew melon (note: many

food theorists suggest eating melons on their own for optimal digestion)

- Mangos, papaya, and kiwis are higher in glycemic index, if that matters to you, as are apples, pears, grapes, and plums. Remember, variety is key, especially in season.
- Kale is the trendy super food
- Green beans
- Broccoli
- Asparagus
- Celery
- Parsley
- Peas (frozen are often best)
- Spinach
- Red peppers (frozen tri-colored slices are available from Trader Joe's)
- Carrots and corn on occasion, or if you have kids and that's all they'll eat.
- Tomatoes
- Tomato sauce jarred – low sodium and low sugar
- Tomatoes chopped, canned, low sodium
- Edamame in shells (frozen)
- Parmesan (real, not filler or processed in the shaker; fresh grated)
- Olive oil
- Spray oil (optional)
- Balsamic vinegar
- Vinaigrette salad dressings (low carb, organic if possible)
- Low sodium V8 (learn to love it!)

- Thin-crust frozen pizza preferably with whole grain crust (read your labels for calories, fat, and sugar. Kashi, Amy's, or California Pizza Kitchen thin-crusts are good in a pinch. Add frozen spinach, kale, and peppers for a more substantial veggie pizza. Sprinkle with Parmesan.)
- Canned soup (veggie based, no cream, low sodium)
- Chicken soup (if you love it)
- Boxed veggie soups (V8 or Imagine)
- Tomato soup (low sodium is best. Add frozen spinach or kale and occasionally a quarter or half cup plain veggie pasta for a quickie dinner.)
- Canned legumes such as chickpeas, black beans, lentils, white beans (low sodium is best)
- Lite soy sauce
- Raw nuts: almonds, cashews, walnuts (bulk or in mini bags from the baking aisle.)
- Dry-roasted peanuts (low salt, if available)
- Hummus (try different flavors; makes a great snack with fresh cut peppers, celery or green beans)
- Sweet potatoes (limit to once or twice a month)
- Quinoa (a high-protein grain; another trendy superfood)
- Barley
- Brown rice
- Whole grain pasta (spinach or tri-colored, and not more than once or twice a month)
- Scandinavian bran crisp-bread

- Steel cut oats (best; in a pinch, go for instant oatmeal packets in plain or low sugar flavors)
- Herbal teas (fruit, green, or mint)

If you must:
- Whole grain or rye bread or thin crackers (be careful here!)
- Fiber rich, low sugar cereal such as Fiber One or plain Total
- Low-fat milk (soy and almond milks can be high in sugar)
- Low-fat cottage cheese in single servings. (Try eating half at a time.)
- Low-fat yogurt. Check labels- sugar and carbs not to exceed 14-16g.

Quick take-away:
Fresh vegetables and fruits are always optimal choices, but it's good to have frozen options on hand when in need.

CHAPTER 13

Reading Labels

IN AN IDEAL world, we would eat fresh, whole food, prepared in a way that keeps it closest to its natural state. But that doesn't always work in the real world. Sometimes we're on the go and short on time. Maybe we don't cook all that well, yet we want to try a variety of foods. And really, all the time we want to eat yummy, fulfilling, tasty, good food.

These days, food manufacturers have created a plethora of convenience foods available in a container or box. Unfortunately, they typically contain preservatives in order to maintain their shelf-life so they can be available at our beck and call. These preservatives foil our desire to eat healthy foods. They can foster cravings and play havoc on our digestive system. But since it's not always possible to buy fresh foods in its most whole, natural form, it's time to educate yourself about how to read and understand food packaging labels.

Here are some simple steps to understanding food labels.

First, know your portion size. It's imperative for all

categories of food you eat, and it really matters when you're looking at prepared foods. If a label says the food product contains 300 calories and 7 grams of fat, you might think that's good and eat the whole package... and then discover that the package actually contained two or three portions. Oops. You've just eaten way too much! Calories, fat, sugar and sodium content all matter in proportion to the serving size. If nothing else - KNOW YOUR PORTION SIZE.

But don't stop there. Ingredients really matter. Ideally, a food label will have no more than five ingredients. If there are more, think twice about bringing it home. (It depends how Good you want to Be.)

Remember that the ingredient at the top of the list is the highest percentage contained in your serving. You definitely want the items in the list to be whole foods you recognize. If the food content contains multi-syllable, chemical language, you most likely want to stay away from it. Even if you're considering a splurge like real ice cream, cookies, or cake, you want it to be made from the freshest, most wholesome ingredients.

Beware of grain products such as cereals, pastas, crackers, or breads that claim they're "all natural" or "high fiber." These products often have added sugar, fat, or sodium (salt). Real whole-grain products list "whole grain" as the first ingredient. Remember that there's a difference between "whole wheat flour" and just wheat flour.

Boxed cereals seem to have the most deceptive marketing campaigns. Besides, eating cereal first thing in the morning spikes your glycemic load, causing you to feel hungry again in a short time. Packaged breads and pastas also have deceptive marketing labels on the package. "All natural" and "whole grain" on the front doesn't always hold up when you read the ingredient content. Anything that lasts a long time in the package has preservatives in it.

These days, you can search the Internet for all kinds of food content including some brand name restaurant's food. Starbucks' website has their drink menu calorie, fat, and sugar contents available. You can also find a list of domestic and imported beers by brand, so you can learn whether that light beer is really worth it in terms of calories and carbohydrates. Search your particular favorite names brand foods or restaurant chains. You'll be amazed at the nutritional content available at your fingertips.

There are a few acceptable packaged foods, such as roasted red peppers, artichoke hearts, sardines, or white meat tuna packed in water (not tuna packed in oil, which is generally cheaper. And, if you're in a restaurant and you order a tuna fish sandwich, which type of tuna do you think they buy in bulk? Just say no!)

Again, the ideal is to eat natural foods closest to their most natural form, which is not in a box or package with a label on it. As food writer Michael Pollan is frequently quoted, "If it was grown *on* a plant, not made *in* a plant, then you can keep it in your kitchen." Speaking of which, I highly recommend Michael Pollan's book, *In Defense of Food: an Eater's Manifesto.*

Quick take-away:
Know the recommended portion size of all packaged foods. Seek out prepared foods containing no more than five ingredients, with a whole food listed first on the label. Don't be fooled by marketing such as "all natural," "whole grain," and "high fiber."

CHAPTER 14

Portion Control

I CAN EASILY gain weight eating healthy food. How? By eating too much.

As I've said repeatedly throughout this book, portion control, choosing wisely, and Being Good to Be Bad helps balance out The Marshall Plan lifestyle: to eat, drink, and look good. If you like to eat out often, as my husband and I do, restaurant dining is the biggest culprit to sabotage your good intentions. It's no secret that portions in restaurants are often ridiculously large and, even at home, we can unknowingly eat too much.

I hope by now you know the one food you get to eat all you want of is GREEN FOOD, (a.k.a. green vegetables,) which should make up two thirds of your plate during lunch and dinner, and even breakfast, if you're so inclined. It's similar to a concept called *volumetrics*, designed by Dr. Barbara Rolls, PhD, where by you crowd out heavier, high-calorie foods by filling up on water-based foods such as green, non-starchy vegetables and soup broths. As I've said, low sodium V8 is a quickie filler to have on hand.

Whether it's meat, poultry, or seafood, three to four ounces is the recommended portion size, which is about the diameter of your palm. A spoonful of oil or salad dressing is about the size of your thumb. Portion size alters in relation to your size: a petite woman requires a smaller portion than a larger man. And in most cases of meat, be it steak or pork, trimming the fat is essential to a healthy cut as well as portion size.

You rarely get a small serving while eating out, so it's important to recognize how much you're eating. I've had one serving of trout consist of two pieces about the size from my hand to my elbow. Crazy! Granted, trout is thin, but that could easily feed two people, and it was too much for one meal.

I often buy a piece of grilled salmon from Whole Foods. It just never tastes the same when I cook it and, on Mondays, I'm in a hurry for lunch. A few months ago I had an inkling the portions were getting really large. Over the holidays I got a new digital food scale that calculates food content. Whoa - my "healthy" piece of salmon for lunch weighed over 7 ounces, with about 440 calories, 20 grams of fat, and 55 grams of protein. That's nutritional value for two meals! Even though it's a healthy choice, it's just too much of a good thing. I cut it in half.

For whole grains, measure a quarter cup of uncooked grain for a single serving and measure a half cup uncooked for whole-grain pasta. It's important to do this exercise to get the visual so when you're served too large a portion you have a good esstimate of how much to eat – and how much to put in a doggie bag to take home.

Can you eat three or four new potatoes rather than a whole baked potato? Can you pull off some of the extra rice when you're having sushi? Can you take off one piece of bread from your sandwich?

Don't throw back handfuls of nuts; even raw nuts contain dense calorie and fat, even though it's good fat. Cut back to a quarter cup serving or, better yet, count your 7-10 nuts and call it a day.

Oftentimes we overeat because it's there. If you eat seven nuts, stop and ask yourself, am I still hungry? If yes, eat a few more, but tune in to see if you're really still hungry. This holds true with every serving of food. Even in a restaurant, you can cut your food in half and check in to see how you feel after the first half. It's nice to take home leftovers for the next day.

Of course when paying for fine dining we tend to eat everything, and really, that's understandable; that's part of our entertainment. But it doesn't hurt to get into the habit of checking in to see if you're truly still hungry. The same holds true with desserts - can you eat just a taste? I can't, but when I do order it (which is rarely), I know I'm going for it and will Be extra Good the week following, and most likely planned for the Being Bad splurge the week prior.

This section is really about MINDFUL EATING. Eat slowly. Savor the flavors and enjoy the food you are eating. Be aware of what you are consuming.

Quick take-away:

Be mindful of portion sizes. Eat half of whatever it is and check in asking yourself, am I really still hungry?

CHAPTER 15

Calories In, Calories Out

CALORIES IN, CALORIES out is a very controversial topic among theorists in the healthy eating world. It makes sense that you consume calories as fuel, and based on your metabolic output, you burn calories. If you want to lose weight or even maintain your current weight, you have to be cognizant of how many calories you're consuming, and roughly understand how many calories you burn. When *guesstimating*, and that's all you can do, overestimate the calories you consume, and underestimate the calories you think you are burning.

The argument to *calories in, calories out* is that aside from age, build, and metabolic rate, the types of calories you consume matter, and there are ways to optimize your metabolism to burn calories. The Marshall Plan is a simple guide to eat, drink, and look good, so if you're interested, you'll have to research the types of intense workouts that increase your metabolic rate.

As I said, the types of calories in this discussion matter. Throughout this book, we've talked about choosing nutrient-dense food. One hundred calories from a slice of avocado is more nutrient-dense than 100 calories from a slice of bread. In general, lean protein choices metabolize more efficiently than carbohydrate calories. Good carbs like whole grains, metabolize better than processed carbohydrates and sugar that turns to fat. Saturated and trans fats go right to your hips while monounsaturated fats aid in digestion; your body needs them.

Never one to be too rigid or strict, I highly recommend you learn about calorie content in the foods you eat. Get a close estimate on your recommended daily caloric intake. Understanding calories per serving (portion sizes) will help you understand why you won't necessarily lose weight eating healthy food. It's so easy to eat too much.

There are several apps and websites to help you estimate your calorie consumption and output. One of my favorites is My Plate on www.Livestrong.com. This tool calculates the number of calories required for your age, weight, activity level, and desired weight with an easy online food diary control. The program contains many name-brand foods, and with regular use you'll learn what foods they list that are closest to the foods you eat. Remember, though, it's an estimate. Over-estimate the calories you consume, and underestimate the calories you burn during exercise.

Once you create an account, log in your current weight, your desired weight, and how many pounds a week you want to lose (one to one and a half pounds per week is realistic). Then every day, record what you eat for each meal. If you eat a salad with assorted toppings, you need to log in the items and amounts separately. You also log in your physical activity; as you burn calories, you're allotted more calories to consume.

Most items listed are an estimate, not actual, but you really can get an idea of how big portion sizes are and how many calories you are consuming and burning. Even if you are only a little obsessive about details, eventually you'll be counting seven raw cashews rather than tossing back a handful. If you're a drinker, you'll learn why I recommend clear alcoholic beverages, and why Being Good to Be Bad is an essential element in successfully changing your lifestyle habits. It's simple: if you eat smart choices and stay within your daily caloric amount, you'll lose weight. I go back to this tool time and time again, especially when I have an upcoming event or over-indulged a little more so than usual. Being Good isn't always easy.

My Plate will also shed light on carbohydrate and fat content, as well as sodium and cholesterol consumption, if you care. However, My Plate does not discern between good carbs, bad carbs or good fat or bad fat. Every body is different, and you'll learn what types of food and nutritional value suits your body and lifestyle needs. Note: caloric needs vary among individuals. If you're trying to lose more than 10 to 30 pounds, please consult your physician before going on a calorie-restricted meal plan.

The moral of this story: you need to learn roughly how many calories you're consuming, because otherwise you can slow weight loss and even gain weight by eating too much of a healthy thing. What you eat affects your weight loss, good or bad.

Move

Now let's talk about *calories out*. Without getting too technical, your body burns different types of calories, at different rates all day long, and it changes depending on age.

Bottom line, ya know ya gotta move, right? And for many of us, at some point in time, doing what we always did doesn't work any more. That being said, you've got to shake it up. Try something different; diversity matters in exercise just the same as with the food you eat. If you stick to running five days a week, your metabolism plateaus and your metabolic rate slows. You effectively burn less calories. Mix it up!

Cross training means diversifying your exercise. You really need to think about finding some way to move every day. For some, you get in the car, drive to work, sit at a desk, drive home at night, and sit on a couch. That's rough for sure. But now you know, movement is a necessity.

Walking is the easiest type of movement to incorporate into your daily routine. When driving to work, the grocery store, a restaurant, or the mall, park far away and walk. Taking an escalator? Walk up as it moves. Given the option, try walking up two to four flights of stairs. At lunch time, go for a walk. You can walk roughly one mile in 20 minutes, so even if you're short on time, walk ten minutes one direction, and ten minutes back. You don't need workout gear for this effort (except for reasonably comfortable shoes), which is especially good if you travel a lot for work and have a tight schedule. Don't let the amount of time available keep you from moving.

Many of you know you have to move more, and you know that breaking a sweat is good for you. Find exercises you like, whether it's long, brisk walks or runs, if that suits you, inside a gym or outside.

After having a baby in July, my dental hygienist's husband and sister-in-law signed her up for a half marathon with six months to train. Sounds like a conspiracy, right? She didn't have time to go to the gym to train x number of miles nor minutes per week. I suggested she get a runner's baby stroller and get out whenever she had time, be it ten, fifteen or thirty minutes. Run 'til you don't want to run anymore, then walk. Feeling recovered? Try running again. Don't worry about time or how long the intervals are, just get started. Eventually she was up to 45 minutes running with the stroller and was motivated to have her husband babysit while she tried longer intervals. In the beginning, start gradually and add on.

My husband and I walk for lunch on the weekends. At first, we'd walk a mile or two, eat lunch (he'd have a beer or two), then walk back. Voila! We knocked off four miles each weekend day. Then, as our infamous Hawaii trip loomed after my 50th birthday, we started walking further – sometimes up to three and a half miles each way. We're crazy walkers, or as our building's concierge calls us, walkaholics. In major cities like New

York City, London, and Hong Kong, to name a few, we've clocked up to 15 miles in a day. One time in LA, yes, that's Los Angeles, the horror city of the motor freeway, we walked 18 miles throughout the day. Crazy, but it helps keep the party pounds off when traveling.

In addition to walking when you can, find other ways of cross-training that you love. Indoor or outdoor cycling, elliptical machines or stair climbers, yoga, Pilates, Zumba, and the increasingly popular "barre" type classes are all designed to help you move and tone you up. Muscle mass burns more calories than fat, so as you add muscle, you increase your metabolism too.

Many of you who have worked out all along may be finding that what you've always done doesn't work as well, so you may be inclined to work out more. The unpleasant truth is that aging plays a factor, causing stress on joints and ligaments which can lead to injury. There is a point in life when too much movement or certain kinds of movement are no longer beneficial to your good health.

About a year after my long term career ended, (and I had a little too much extra time to workout,) an old hamstring injury reared its ugly head. I was in a lot of pain and could barely stand on one leg when a woman in my gym recommended acupuncture. For my first appointment with Dr. He, I had a list of all the activities I did during the week; at nearly 52 years old I felt rather accomplished with my lifelong physical fitness regime.

When I told him I could barely stand on one leg, he stared blankly into my eyes. "Why do you want to do that?" he inquired. "Yoga!" I boasted. He paused, and proceeded to lecture me on the virtues of *finding the window*. "You are not 20. You must find the window of activity that is balanced for your age. You can fight Mother Nature, but she will always win." As my mobility increased, he encouraged me to find the window of activity that was "healthy" for my body. The old adage, *less is more* prevails.

It may seem counterintuitive to work out less and find more diverse things to do. This is where smart food choices come into play. It's a difficult balance, especially if you sometimes feel more hungry because of a regular or aggressive work out routine.

Yet another seemingly contradictory recommendation: sleep matters more than working out. Let's say you're trying to add movement to your daily routine. With a hectic schedule, you decide to wake up early to get in some kind of workout. Commendable indeed, and I mean that seriously. It's worth the extra effort, but listening to your body is the most important factor. The Marshall Plan is far from bootcamp. If you're tired, sleep in one day. Maybe consider going to bed earlier, or take a 10-20 minute nap in the afternoon or early evening. This doesn't mean forgo all your commitments to get up early to get in your workout. This means you're tuned in and listening to your body's needs.

When you have erratic sleep, your body produces the hormone cortisol, which can cause you to store belly fat (gasp, abhor) despite all your good intentions. Besides, sleep is the most critical medicine for living a healthy, vital life, fighting off signs of aging and disease.

Studies are inconclusive whether working out

decreases or stimulates appetite. You have to tune in and determine for yourself. If what you've always done isn't working, odds are working out stimulates your appetite and you have to watch what you eat afterwards. Also, be wary of calorie-burning counts on electronic equipment like treadmills, stairclimbers, ellipticals, etc. Unless you wear a heart rate monitor that calculates your age, height, and weight, you most likely burn LESS than stated on the machine's calorie count.

The biggest trap in working out is you *think you deserve* to eat more because you worked out. If you're trying to manage your weight or lose a few pounds, you'll sabotage your success by overeating after working out. I know people who actually gained weight after starting an exercise regime because they overestimated calories burned and underestimated calories consumed after a workout.

Quick take-away:
Find movement you enjoy, and do something every day.

Metabolism cha-cha-cha-changes in your 40s and 50s

What use to work to manage our weight or stay in our skinny jeans just stops working. Men and women alike experience slowing metabolism in their 40s and 50s. For some women, it starts in their 30s and can be linked to child bearing.

Is it normal? Heck yes, but it isn't hopeless to the point of nothing you can do about it. True, most of us will never return to our first driver's license weight, but we can all make an effort to do better.

If you're not motivated by skinny jeans, eating better for your good health and longevity should matter. As one of my favorite clients said, she "just didn't want to eat like a sixteen-year-old any longer." It's time to become aware, intelligent even, about healthy food. You can train your tastebuds to like green vegetables, less salt, less fat, less bad carbohydrates, and less sugar.

Remember, we're not saying you can never eat seemingly "bad" foods again. We're just saying that by changing your overall lifestyle eating habits, you make healthy good food the norm, and the delicious bad stuff is the exception.

I never said it was easy, but it is doable, and it can be a gradual process where you determine how aggressively you want to change. That's the secret to long-term success in a lifestyle change versus a short-term diet. To be cliché about it, it's a journey, not a destination, and that really is the truth. You just gotta want it!

Quick take-away:
Know your requirements to help you meet your goals. When estimating your intake, overestimate the calories you consume, and underestimate the calories you think you are burning.

CHAPTER 16

Weighing In

To WEIGH OR not to weigh, this is a heavily debated question. Many experts claim you should not weigh yourself because you'll get too hung up on numbers. On the other hand, if you're trying to lose weight for a specific event or goal, weighing in gives you a motivating visual.

In our mid-forties and up, our metabolism slows and our pants get tight. Many of us give in to larger pants instead of giving up some overeating habits. During my mid-forties I tried not weighing in and not being too hung up on the numbers. As a result, I gave in to a larger pants size, giving credence to the possibility that middle-age metabolic change took it out of my control.

To some extent it's true. During middle age, the body does change. Added inches creep up around your waist, and they might seem out of your control, yet weight fluctuation calls for a change in eating and movement behavior. So, in my view, there is value in watching your numbers, along with portion control and calorie intake.

If you choose to weigh in, the key is to weigh yourself at the same time of day. I also like to check in on the same days of the week, typically Wednesday and Friday. I weigh in on Wednesday after two days of Being Good to decrease party pounds from the weekend. By Friday, I hope to be at the week's lowest going into the weekend. If I'm as low as I'd like, I might choose to splurge and order sweet potato fries. If I'm not as low as expected on Friday, I hesitate before sneaking that french fry off my husband's plate.

The number on Wednesday determines the level of Good required that week for me to be Bad again the following weekend. You know how it goes, right? And at any weigh-in I might have an eye-opener – I might be higher than I anticipated. That means I have to be more Good than Bad over the next few days, weekend or not. It's even happened that I'm lower than I expected, and then I treat myself to a guilt free splurge.

Naturally your weight fluctuates based on the time of day, what you're wearing, food consumption, or water weight, and surely you know that different scales tell different tales. Therefore it's a good idea to weigh yourself at the same time of day on the same scale. It is most likely no surprise I weigh myself first thing in the morning. It's about setting a benchmark and understanding how your weight fluctuates around your goals.

It's important to give yourself a high and low range for desired weight. This compensates for water-weight fluctuations, and it's an easy way to set goals, whether you want to stair-step your weight lower, or just maintain your desired weight. The range can be two or three pounds for women, or up to five pounds for men.

For me, my satisfaction depends on how those damn skinny jeans fit. Develop your own quirky gauge, but set your limits. That way, as the numbers creep up, you can spot it, own it, and say "whoa, it's time to amp up the Being Good part." Gaining one to two pounds over a weekend is not a big deal for a woman, but if you're not good during the week, it can creep up to two or three pounds or more, by the end of the month. For men, a fluctuation of two to three pounds is not a big deal, but anything over that is a warning sign.

Weighing in doesn't have to be obsessive; keep a realistic perspective. Don't worry about whether muscle weighs more than fat. If you're gaining muscle weight, good for you, your clothes will fit looser. Typically most of us still have a little fat to lose.

Happy Monday!

So you lost a few pounds Being Good to Be Bad last week, and now you're on the other side of Bad and it was so worth it.

The best thing about The Marshall Plan is it's a *lighthearted* guide for staying slim and having fun. The Marshall Plan is about never feeling guilty or beating yourself up, because that wouldn't be fun, would it? Don't be disillusioned, when you enjoy eating, weight gain can be cyclical – three steps forward, two steps back.

Every day offers an opportunity for a fresh start to offset any indulgence that occurred over the weekend or a holiday. Any day is a good time to reflect on the areas of eating you can do better next time, and it's great to savor those bites of chocolate mousse cake because you know you won't have it again for a while.

Monday through Wednesday or Thursday is the time to set your strongest intent to follow The Marshall Plan guidelines for eating to look and feel good. The new day is the greatest day to offset fun splurges or excess, especially when eating out, traveling, or not working out regularly.

Mindful eating, smart choices, portion control, and movement are keys to success when balancing eating to look and feel good, and having fun!

Quick take-away:
Weigh in. At some point, living la vida loca (the crazy life) catches up with you. Today is the first day of the rest of your life. Yes, it sounds hokey but it's so darn true. Take charge of your eating habits for a longer, healthier, happier lifestyle.

CHAPTER 17

Satisfying Good Food - The Whole Food Movement

By NOW YOU'VE probably recognized a theme interwoven throughout the lifestyle change in The Marshall Plan. Not only do we gotta eat, we want to eat! You want to enjoy eating all the time, without overindulging and threatening your health. You want to feel good and look good, living to your optimal good health potential.

Being Good doesn't mean punishment. You want to eat yummy, healthy food most of the time. And you absolutely want to treat yourself to something indulgent when you decide it's the right time, whether on the weekend, a vacation, or special occasion.

Satisfying, good food means good quality, thoughtfully-prepared meals. Fortunately, there's a huge movement calling for fresh food farm to table. Many grocery stores, including some Walmart stores, feature sections of locally grown fruits and vegetables. Meat and poultry has entered the game with organic or grass-fed offerings, versus hormone-infused, mass-produced and processed.

And now we get into an increasingly gray area which might surprise you: buying organics. Eating good food has become so trendy that food manufacturers slap organic labels on everything. Fortunately, there are FDA guidelines regulating organic food labeling. In short, organic packaged foods refers not only to the food itself, but how it is produced, grown, and processed. If you're interested, you can research more on organic farming and regulations.

When buying organic fruits and vegetables, there are two lists that offer guidelines on what's good, what's bad. The lists actually fluctuate seasonally, so check the Internet for the most recent version of the Dirty Dozen and the Clean Fifteen. In general, fruits or vegetables that have a thick, removable skin, are less likely to be affected by pesticides. The Clean Fifteen exemplifies choices that do *not* need to be organic.

The Clean Fifteen:
— onions
— sweet corn
— pineapples
— avocado
— cabbage
— sweet peas
— asparagus
— mangoes
— eggplant
— kiwi
— domestic cantaloupe
— sweet potatoes

- grapefruit
- watermelon
- bananas

The Environmental Working Group recommends choosing organic when buying The Dirty Dozen fruits and veggies that have thinner skins that are easier for chemicals to penetrate.

The Dirty Dozen Plus:
- apples
- celery
- sweet bell peppers
- peaches
- strawberries
- imported nectarines
- grapes
- spinach
- lettuce
- cucumbers
- domestic blueberries
- potatoes
- green beans
- kale, collards, and leafy greens

Unfortunately, some grocery markets take advantage of this increased popularity in organics by increasing the price. A pint of organic strawberries in season from the exact same farm can be $1.49 more than the non-organic pint. While it's true that organic farming can be more costly (at least initially) for the farmers, that still seems like an exceedingly high difference, yet there are more and more studies about contaminated berries. You really must decide for yourself. Keep a list of the Dirty Dozen and Clean Fifteen (there's an app for that,) and be mindful of your choices when grocery shopping.

Then we get into the discussion of local food, which typically means the fruit and vegetables are trucked in less than 100 miles. Many organic fruits and vegetables are flown in from South America, Asia, or the opposite coast from you.

So which is better? In my circle of health aficionados, we are trending toward choosing local foods, whether organic or not, over organic foods flown in from around the world. And remember, when eating out, you have no control over which components of your meal are organic or not, and you'll make yourself (and your significant other and friends) crazy trying to be too rigid about this.

Buried in this debate is the issue of seasonal fruits and vegetables. Not long ago, living in the Midwest meant you could only get strawberries, blueberries, and peaches (for instance) in the warmer summer months. I remember making my favorite summer salad with fresh peaches as often as possible because I knew by the end of August, peach season would be over and I'd have to wait until next year to devour it again.

Nowadays, you can get fresh melons and berries of all varieties throughout the year. But have you noticed that they don't always taste that good, especially in November through February? And the price of asparagus in the winter is sky high because it comes from South America.

In a way, it's a luxurious problem to have: easy access to whatever we want when we want it. But the price we pay is greater than financial; we pay the price in lack of flavor, and nutrients. Do I eat only seasonal choices as nature planned it? Not always, but I do make an effort to seek out seasonal fruits and vegetables. Sautéed swiss chard is cooked the same way as sautéed spinach or bok choy, so it's not really that complicated, and I'm diversifying my nutrient content. It's not hard to identify seasonal fruits and vegetables. In the produce department, stop. Look around. Seasonal fruits and vegetables are typically prominently featured in abundance, and often on promotion.

Quick take-away: Local is best; you don't need to buy organic fruit or vegetables with skin on, and seek out new varieties of seasonal fare.

Cravings - You Can Train Your Brain

There is a lot of talk in the media these days about food addiction. I'm certainly not going to judge the validity of extreme cases, but in general, we have the power to alter our taste preferences and learn to enjoy eating fresh whole foods.

Cravings aren't just psychological. If you eat sugar-laden foods, your body craves more sugar. Same holds true for artificial sweeteners and salt. So, can you train your brain and body to crave green food? Yes.

Awareness is the key to any change. You have to tune in and detect what triggers your desire for certain foods. For some, it's a mere glance at a clock. Three o'clock means M&Ms or something sweet, whether it's candy, juice or soda. For others, it means salty snacks. Let's face it, women learn early on, what weeks of the month bingeing on sweet snacks is justified. And as we know by now, excess sugar turns to fat.

If you love chocolate, choose rich, dark chocolate versus milk chocolate. Just think, eating half or even a whole dark organic chocolate bar is a better choice than cookies, candies, or fudge bars. Savor the bites, however many.

Raw nuts are a super food, and a scant quarter cup (about 10 nuts) is a healthy, nutrient-dense snack. If you love salty foods, you can wean yourself off of salted nuts to raw nuts in simple stages. Begin mixing raw nuts with your favorite roasted, salted nuts, gradually adding more raw, unsalted nuts and fewer roasted, salted nuts to the mix. Eventually, you'll enjoy a healthy, protein-packed snack of raw nuts. Remember to note the portion size; it's really important here, because if you throw back handfuls of any nuts, raw or other, you'll be consuming too much fat. Eat your nuts one at a time and savor the flavor. Unsalted, dry-roasted peanuts are a good alternative choice.

The same holds true for healthy, whole foods. In the greens section, we discussed how to wean off butter-laden sauces and creamy dressings. Once you make the switch and incorporate whole, fresh, glorious green food into several meals each day, you'll notice a green-food craving when you neglect your intake. (If you live in Atlanta, try Souper Jenny's Super Power Green vegan soup, an orgasmically delicious addiction.)

When traveling, it can be strangely challenging to get good green food. We travel overnight to visit my husband's family in the English countryside. We eat a relatively healthy dinner on board and typically skip the morning meal service. It's really too short a time between meals to warrant a whole breakfast, and usually the choices are fat ladened eggs and sausages served with croissant or bagel. Even the side of crispy, tasteless fruit in unappealing.

When we arrive at his mum's house early afternoon, cheese (and butter if you want) sandwiches on white bread or biscuits are the fare – and I feel psycho for green vegetables by mid-afternoon. At the pub next door I settle for carrots with a few sprigs of broccoli. You wouldn't think it's so difficult to get green vegetables in a whole 24-hour period, but I was ready to chomp on a bush outside (although at Christmas, they were covered in snow).

Similar situations hold true in organized business meetings. Green food is not the norm as it should be. (Remember, iceberg lettuce doesn't count.)

The point is, you can wean yourself off unhealthy cravings and create new ones. This is not to say you never indulge in sweets or salty treats. Heck no! Deprivation is NOT part of The Marshall Plan. When you indulge, go for the good stuff, and be aware that it is the exception, not the norm. If you notice any triggers in the days that follow an indulgence, be aware and just say no. Remind yourself that delectable treat will always be available another time.

Quick take-away:
You have to wean yourself off addictive, processed foods. You can train your tastebuds and your brain to enjoy healthy, fresh, whole food choices.

CHAPTER 18

Diversity Matters

AS WITH EVERYTHING in life, and as I've said repeatedly in this book, diversity matters.

Let's make sure we understand what this means in context.

di·ver·si·ty

1. the state or fact of being diverse; difference; unlikeness.

2. variety; multiformity.

—Synonyms - change, difference, variation, dissimilarity.

In the case of food, variety is key; that means "mix it up." My former style of eating was more of a monoculture: when I found something I liked, I ate it many days a week. It was also simple, literally a "no brainer" when planning meals and grocery shopping.

This behavior was true whether "dieting" or

supposedly eating healthy, but it's not good for your metabolism or nutritional intake.

It may take a little more time and thought to diversify your consumption, but you're better off for it. That's why we call it *mindful eating*. Eating the same thing every day is just not good for you. You need to diversify to get a variety of nutrients – and it's not enough to say you're taking vitamin supplements. There are so many micronutrients in foods that we're just not aware of and couldn't possibly supplement, even if we did understand how they all interact.

Breakfast

It's not cliché. Breakfast is the most important meal of the day.

Let's break it down: you haven't eaten for eight to 12 hours and you need to break that fast. You must fuel your body. Skipping this important meal slows your metabolism. Eating breakfast within the first hour after waking *boosts your metabolism*.

Many people eat breakfast on the run. You often hear people talk about consuming a banana per day, a pack of instant oatmeal, a yogurt, or, worse, a yogurt smoothie. With these choices, you're likely to be consuming too much sugar, especially first thing in the morning after your system has had an eight-hour-plus fast.

High sugar and high carbohydrate choices race through your system. You'll be hungry sooner. On the other hand, eating protein first thing in the morning helps boost your metabolism and stave off hunger. Three, antioxidant rich walnuts with a big glass of water on an empty stomach will balance your blood sugar.

Other theories suggest eating only fruit until noon for a cleansing ritual. Personally, I eat fresh fruit about 30 minutes after the walnuts. Once in a blue moon, I'll have single servings of low fat cottage cheese on hand and, although theories suggest eating fruit on its own, I love cottage cheese and fruit. It's a childhood favorite. What about adding protein powder to a fresh fruit smoothie? While you are achieving the protein, you're also adding a processed food. In moderation, a few times a month or when on the go, it is okay. If you're buying a 16-ounce smoothie from a shop, can you drink half? Yes, it's wasteful, but the calories really add up.

As discussed, dairy is a controversial food category. Many people eat low-fat yogurt as a healthy choice, but if you check the sugar content, you may find it's doing more harm than good. Greek yogurt is a better option, but not every day. Can you cut it down to two to three times per week? And once you get there, can you cut it down to one or two times a month? Again, can you shift the portion size to a dollop of yogurt on a bowl of fruit rather than eating an entire container of yogurt at one meal. It's the same if you love milk: drink a glass now and then, just not every day. In general, reducing dairy is a good idea. We're talking about one to two times per month, not as a daily staple or weekly.

Remember diversity matters so don't eat the same thing every day. One of my winter favorites is almond butter on whole grain toast or bran crisp-bread. Other days it might be a slice of avocado or smoked salmon on a bran crisp-bread. Occasionally, I'll scramble eggs or tofu with sautéed vegetables. On the run, prepare hard boiled eggs the night before.

Slow-cooking steel-cut oats is the healthiest whole grain choice, but not always the most convenient. You can make a large batch once a week, scoop out a half-cup serving, add a little water, and microwave. Voila! You have steel cut oats in less than a minute; add antioxidant rich cinnamon and a few chopped raw nuts for protein. In a hurry, add the same to a half packet of plain, instant oatmeal to start your day.

Depending on your creative cooking skills, the choices really are endless. These are just my "fast food" staples.

More Reasons Diversity Matters....

There are many arguments on behalf of vegan eating; I've "been there, tried that," but truth is if you dine out in restaurants, it's difficult to control hidden dairy, along with sugar, fat, and salt, (not to be a killjoy). But my real struggle with vegan eating is that I love cheese. I reserve my dairy intake for sharing a really good cheese plate while dining out somewhere yummy. I also love an occasional serving of low-fat cottage cheese with fruit for breakfast, or on a baked sweet potato for dinner. For me, vegan eating is too rigid. It's highly beneficial for many people. You decide.

Tofu, typically considered a "health" food, is a derivative from soy. It's a vegetarian source of high protein and healthy fat. It can be blended into smoothies, scrambled with veggies, or tossed in soups or salads. I love the texture and the way it absorbs whatever flavors you choose to create through spices and sauces. I could eat it two or three times a day, every day. So imagine my dismay when I learned that too much tofu can slow your metabolism and even have toxic effects.

Soy is sometimes promoted to peri-menopausal women to ease some of the annoying symptoms. But most soy is genetically modified and grown in huge crops due to its popularity. Some reports claim GMO soy negatively affects thyroid, especially in a processed state like bars, cereals, and milk. Also, when you read your labels, soy products, particularly soy milk, tend to have a lot of added sugar.

In short, over-consumption of over-processed genetically modified soy can be toxic. Soy, in its most natural state, is still a good source of lean protein; so again, everything in moderation.

This philosophy holds true for meats, poultry, and seafood. Grass-fed beef and free-range poultry are popular both for the more natural feed and more humane treatment on the farm and at the time of slaughter. Always select lean cuts of meat like filet steak and white sections of pork and poultry.

There's a lot of controversy over fresh fish and mercury levels, unnatural dyes in farmed fish, and cholesterol in shellfish. Omega 3-rich, fresh salmon is still one of your best bets - heavens, I hope so because I eat it several times a week. (See, there I go again, finding something I like that's healthy and eating it regularly. Mix it up - diversity matters!) Because of its popularity, salmon is often farmed and dyed to achieve that fresh pink color. In some regular grocery stores, that's all you can get.

Speak up! Tell the people behind the counters that you don't want dyed salmon; tell the store manager. There will be a time when much of the fish we eat is farmed, and many farmers are using sustainable practices. Nonetheless, they don't have to dye it.

You can check online for eco fish selections – those not overly fished or with high mercury levels. If you diversify your selection, you shouldn't have to worry all that much, but if you eat a lot of fish, it's good to know what kinds are better for you.

Sometimes I like to open the fridge and see what's randomly left in there and make what I call a "refrigerator picnic salad." It's often a fun and flavorful mix of unexpected combinations. One time it was just a peach, red pepper, and avocado. Sometimes it's mango, asparagus, and zucchini. All of it sounds good. Try it... mix it up.

Here's another reason diversity matters. One evening, my husband called me saying I'd be proud he went to the doctor that day. My eyes widened in terror because he doesn't go to a doctor unless I make him. He had been feeling discomfort from indigestion for a few weeks, so initiating his own trip to the doctor meant he really wasn't feeling well.

For simplicity's sake, my husband would eat the same thing Monday through Thursday in an effort to Be Good so he could Be Bad on the weekend. His monoculture diet consisted of grilled Springer Mountain chicken breast, frozen or steamed fresh peas, broccoli, brussels sprouts, or cauliflower. The good news: the lean protein, lots of vegetables, and low carbohydrate meal plan helped him maintain his desired weight. The bad news: after eight to twelve months eating these same cruciferous, stalky vegetables, he developed severe gastric indigestion.

He's since switched to soft green vegetables and mixed a variety of seafood into the weekly diet, because even chicken breast is slightly more difficult to digest. This meant giving his meal plan more attention and, to his regret, going to the grocery store more often. As you might imagine, I'd been suggesting he mix it up for months, but I never dreamed he could develop such a severe condition.

Through training, research, and experience, I've learned that diversifying the foods I eat, making certain they are tasty and satisfying, makes it easy to maintain my desired weight. As a result, I've been able to enjoy a guilt free splurge (or two or three) along the way. Once you add diversity to your lifestyle, you won't find yourself succumbing to bingeing and unwanted weight gain. Even while traveling, the weight gain pendulum isn't as extreme as when I tried to "diet" during the week, and gorged on the weekend.

Quick take-away:
Diversify your food choices for every meal
and snacks too. Mix it up!

Super Foods

As healthy eating grows trendier and trendier, every year there's another list or two of super foods.

Super foods are popularly touted as the most nutrient dense, vitality nourishing, cancer preventing, memory boosting keys to living a long, healthy lifestyle. Choosing these foods means getting the "biggest bang for your buck," as my father would say. A lifestyle diet rich in super foods is said to improve your mood, alter or even prevent disease, and slow signs of aging.

Salmon always tops the lists, best known for its lean protein and heart-healthy, cholesterol-reducing, Omega 3 antioxidants. Walnuts have similar properties. Kale and quinoa (pronounced kin-wa,) are protein-rich super foods, as are antioxidant-packed organic blueberries, fresh or frozen. Deep-colored vegetables make the super food list, as do fiber-rich legumes cooked simply.

The antioxidants in green tea promote healthy metabolism, as does deep, dark chocolate, made with 60-70% cocoa beans (it has less sugar and fat than other chocolate). Some lists include a glass of red wine. Now there's a combo, 2-3 ounces of red wine and a one-inch square of dark chocolate, yum!

A newscaster recently said, "Move over kale and quinoa, chia seeds are the new super food." A natural food source derivative of the cha cha cha chia plant, chia is part of the mint family from the Salvia Hispanic grown in deserts in Mexico – but you don't need to know all that! What you *do* want to know is that organic chia seeds are high in fiber, balancing your blood sugar and slowing carbohydrate conversion to sugar. Chia seeds are loaded with heart-healthy Omega 3s, as well as protein for lean muscle mass and extended energy. Chia seeds improve digestion and are rich in age-defying antioxidants and calcium, and balance your electrolytes.

It's easy to hear all the benefits and think it's too good to be true, but chia seeds really do offer big bang for your buck. The problem is that it's difficult to get in as much as recommended. I say spoon it on when you can and try harder next time. It doesn't really have much flavor, but it does add texture. You can add it to anything: fruit, veggies, salads, soup, potatoes, popcorn, meat, poultry or fish, ice cream - I mean anything you don't mind adding it too. Me, I sprinkle it on fruit in the morning, then sometimes veggies later in the day. I've sprinkled it on microwave popcorn (fresh, organic, no oil) just because I thought of it. Buy it and try it.

Goji and acai berries and pomegranates in their natural form have been on the super food list for realistic benefits, but the health food industry began manufacturing all kinds of processed foods containing them, which minimizes the impact of their benefits. Skip the processed versions, and if you like fresh pomegranate seeds in your salad, go for it.

It's wise to choose super foods when you have the opportunity. The reasons are simple: heart healthy, lean protein, boost antioxidants, fight free radicals and inflammation, while the fiber-rich super foods keep toxins moving out of your system. On The Marshall Plan, we always want the biggest bang for our buck.

Lists of super foods can vary, so investigate what choices makes sense for you.

Quick take-away:
Choose super foods when given the option.
Salmon, walnuts, quinoa, kale, blueberries, red wine, and dark chocolate top the lists.

Tea Time - afternoon tea

It's not that my English in-laws have gotten to me. My version of afternoon tea is a bit different from theirs. No scones with clotted cream, and the only caffeine is in green tea, which is loaded with antioxidants (and some studies suggest green tea boosts metabolism). Green tea with lemon or mint can cut the bitterness, and it's a great mid-afternoon pick me up. If you can acquire a taste for a more earthy tea, Bancha tea, a form of green tea stems, is loaded with antioxidants and some calcium.

If you tend to crave sweets at night, try a cup of black cherry, red raspberry, orange, or vanilla flavored tea. Mint tea is good for digestion, and chocolate mint tea is tasty, but not quite yummy enough to replace a hot chocolate addict's craving. There are so many unique herbal teas out there, you could spend a small fortune stocking up on assorted varieties. If you want to Be Good, steer away from adding sweetener of any kind, and fill up on herbal tea!

Quick take-away:
Use herbal tea as a no-calorie filler both mid-afternoon and late evenings whether reading, writing, or while watching TV.

CHAPTER 19

Vitamins

It's NEARLY IMPOSSIBLE to get enough vitamins and minerals from food you eat, and it would have to be all natural, all organic, picked fresh, measured quantities, and probably too many calories of food every day. Ain't gonna happen. Fresh produce begins to lose nutrient content the minute it's picked, then transported to a distributor, then transported to the grocery store, then you buy and store what you've bought. Foods no longer contain nutrients levels required for optimal health.

Whether meat, poultry, seafood, fruits, vegetables, nuts, or legumes, diversity matters to get the balanced vitamins and minerals your body needs to operate as a healthy well-oiled machine. Truth is, no matter how vigilant you are making smart choices for food, you just can't be sure that you're getting the recommended daily allotment of vitamins and nutrients. So at minimum, take a multi vitamin; it doesn't have to be every day, just more often than not. In general, there are little risks to taking a multi-vitamin; there are mainly benefits. Your system will have a more balanced intake of vitamins and minerals along with antioxidants that lower the inflammation that causes disease. Note: there are vitamin restrictions for certain "groups," so always consult your primary health care provider before taking new vitamins.

However, even when you take a vitamin, there's no guarantee that you'll actually absorb everything as printed on the label. The FDA does not regulate what goes into vitamins compared to what's on the label, even for all-natural. Of course, natural is better than synthetic. Buy better-quality, all-natural vitamins from a specialty store, rather than what the drugstore has to offer. Timed-release vitamins are a good option.

Yes, it's a guessing game, and there are no guarantees, but as I said, there's also relatively little risk, and many benefits in taking a multi-vitamin. Read your labels and look for ingredients that you're familiar with and appeal to you, whether it's gluten free, iron free, etc. If you're new at this, again, consult your health practitioner.

Surprisingly, most multi-vitamins do not provide the recommended daily allowance for calcium, which is 1000 mg per day. If you eat a reduced-dairy diet, you may want to supplement 500 -1000 mg of calcium daily. Calcium chews are fun if you have a sweet tooth, but you should only eat one. Look for calcium with magnesium for proper absorption. Too much calcium can lead to constipation among other things, and we don't want that.

You can use an extra 1000 mg of vitamin C as an immune system boost, especially in winter, if sick people are around, or you plan to travel. If you take your multi-vitamin after breakfast, take the extra C in the evening, opposite of when you take the multi vitamin. Otherwise you may just eliminate the extra vitamins when you release water. If you feel the symptoms of a cold coming on, boost the dosage to two to three times per day, just for a few days. You don't want to overdose vitamin C either; it can cause stomach upset and diarrhea. Zinc has many of the immune system boosting qualities as vitamin C. Some people take extra vitamin E, not to exceed 500 i.u./day, for antioxidant skincare.

Omega 3-packed fish oil soft-gels help decrease cholesterol, lowering blood triglyceride levels and reducing the risk of heart attack and strokes, lowering blood pressure, and reducing the stiffness and joint tenderness associated with rheumatoid arthritis. Omega 3 fish-oil supplements may also help improve or prevent cancer, Alzheimer's disease and dementia, depression, heart disease, diabetes, and arthritis. Fish oil has also been shown to improve concentration and clearer thinking in general. It's noted to aid in building muscle, losing fat, and improving fitness level or athletic ability in any capacity.

Flaxseed oil also boosts antioxidants, lowers cholesterol, protects against cancer, reduces inflammation, and aids in digestion.

Spirulina is a blend of greens that remove toxins and are an anti-inflammatory. For 500 mg, 6 tablets/day, spirulina is less expensive than blue-green algae, which is also a good option.

Remember to take all vitamins after a meal to avoid nausea.

Proper nutrient balance is as effective as exercise in lowering the inflammation that causes disease. Most of us take supplements in some form based on what we've read or heard. If you're serious – or just seriously confused – about taking vitamins, talk to your health practitioner to determine what's right for you.

You really don't have to go overboard with an assortment of supplements. Once I had a workman in my kitchen who asked if I was a hypochondriac. I said no, and wondered why he asked. He'd noticed I had seven jars of assorted supplements lined up along the wall. At that time I had gone to a kinesiologist who had prescribed a vast assortment of supplements based on a deficiency test. Once I finished them, I reduced my intake. That was over 20 years ago.

Yes, a lot of people suffer from food allergies and would benefit greatly from certain dietary changes in their lives, but for the purpose of The Marshall Plan, we're relatively healthy people who want to do the best we can to look good and feel good without making ourselves crazy.

Quick take-away:
Take a well balanced, natural multi-vitamin
once a day or every other day. Read your
labels to understand what you're getting.

CHAPTER 20

Dining Out

DINING OUT IS the greatest conflict for The Marshall Plan. It can sabotage all your best efforts for Being Good, but it's so much fun! And let's not forget that we're Being Good so we can Be Bad and have fun.

For us, the weekends are rough. My husband likes to eat dinner out Friday and Saturday as well as lunch out Saturday and Sunday. Only recently have I been able to get him to eat dinner in on Sunday nights (and not only do I have to plan it ahead, it needs to be somewhat fun).

The main reason eating out is so dangerous is because you typically eat more calories, even if you order relatively "clean" food. Portion size is a challenge when dining out, especially if it's really tasty food, we tend to eat it all. Going out frequently means trying to Be relatively Good in the Bad environment. Ordering off the menu is all about making smart choices.

Let's start with cocktails. As stated earlier, drink clear liquids beginning with lots of water, be it sparkling or still, bottled or tap. From an environmental position, we try not to drink bottled water when dining out in the U.S. (International water is a different situation.) I like sparkling water occasionally, especially when I'm not indulging in a libation, but note that it can cause bloating or gas. Club soda is another good option, but it contains sodium, causing more bloat.

Which brings me to libations. Many restaurants have festive artsy cocktail menus, but beware, most contain juices and simple syrups which equals SUGAR which equals excess carbs, which equals belly fat. So if you've been exceptionally Good, go ahead and try *one*. Otherwise, if your intention is be moderately Good, save yourself for the weekend and stick to clear liquids: champagne, white wine, lite beer, or vodka and soda. Gin and soda works, only I've yet to meet a gin and tonic drinker who will go for this. They usually have gin on the rocks or gin and diet tonic. Of course, the problem with diet sodas is that the artificial sweeteners fuel sweet cravings.

In my youth I was a vodka and soda gal, so sticking with that or switching to wine or champagne is not a problem. Gin and tonic drinkers, whoa - take heed! It's time to cut out the tonic.

One of our goals is to slow down the dining experience, although it sometimes seems the restaurant's goal is to turn the table as quickly as possible. We order courses one at a time, whether the waiter likes it or not.

If your intent is to splurge, go for it. I don't have to tell anyone how to indulge their eating desires. On the other hand, if you want to be moderately Good, look for "clean" food, meaning lightly grilled and without heavy sauce. Begin by sharing a starter or appetizer. Grilled or sautéed protein like seafood, chicken, or vegetables is a good choice. Only see fried calamari on the menu? Ask for it sautéed.

We will split a cheese plate now and then, and eat it with crusty bread, savoring every morsel. I've eaten bites of a Pablano pepper stuffed with chorizo, again shared. To my delight, I've learned bites of anything won't sabotage The Marshall Plan.

Bread – did you catch it earlier? I did say I enjoy crusty bread. A few rules about bread:

You can just say no to having the breadbasket delivered to your table, providing the other guests are in agreement. And only eat bread that is so delicious on its own, it doesn't need butter to make it better. Some restaurants offer flavored butters, and it's okay to taste a smidge, but stay away from bread that needs butter slathered all over to help it go down. Be on guard in the restaurants that drop single rolls onto your bread plate. When you're not looking, they swoop down and drop off another. When indulging, just eat one.

Next course, share or eat your own mixed greens salad with vinaigrette on the side. It seems like even in better restaurants they douse lettuce in dressing, so it's always safest to add it to your taste. The goal is to crowd out hunger with greens. And remember, no cream-based dressing, including Caesar.

At this point, you might consider ordering a small plate from the appetizer list plus a green vegetable side for your main meal. Try eating your veggies first, again, filling up your stomach. If you really want an entree, order grilled or sautéed chicken, fish, pork chop, or filet mignon, with sauce on the side so you have the option to drizzle on just a smidgen to taste.

Anything baked often comes in sauce. Watch out for buttery or creamy sauces. If your main entrée arrives floating in sauce, move it to another plate such as your bread plate. Panfried seafood or poultry is acceptable when a must, but stay clear of deep fried (unless you're going for fish 'n' chips).

When eating your entree, cut large portions in half, eating only one half. Keep in mind, a 3oz. serving is about the size of the palm of your hand. At this point, check in with yourself; are you really still hungry? Do you really need or want to eat more? If not, share the other half of your entree or take home leftovers if possible. I know, I really hate to waste food, but you have to honor your priorities.

Typically, your entree will come with potato or rice. Ask them to hold the starch – i.e., not even bring it on your plate – and you can guarantee you won't eat it. Stay clear of white rice blends and mashed potatoes; both have a lot of hidden fats as well as processed carbohydrates (empty calories). Choose whole grains when given the option, and remember that sweet or new potatoes are a more nutrient-dense option.

Enjoy french fries if you're going all out. Thicker-cut steak fries absorb less oil than crispy shoestring potatoes; beware of double dipped french fries.

Dessert? It's entirely up to you. You can look for lighter choices here too. Cakes, tortes, ice cream, and creme brûlée are high in calories, sugar, and bad fat. Sorbet has less bad fat. If you're going to indulge, make it worthwhile, share, and enjoy. If a friend insists on ordering a dessert to share, I let her make the choice in hopes she picks something I'm less interested in, so I'll eat less of it.

Another good tip for eating out is to not go out starving. Sometimes I'll have chopped red pepper, green veggies, a cup of pureed green vegetable soup, or low-sodium V8 before dining out to stave off hunger pangs and prevent diving into the bread basket when I get there.

If you're eating breakfast or brunch out, watch omelets and even scrambled eggs when dining out. Unknown and usually excess amounts of butter and milk are added; the fluffier the more dangerous. Try to keep it to two-egg servings; many omelets are three to four eggs so try eating just half. Watch out for fatty meats like bacon or sausage, and creamy cheese fillings.

Love eggs benedict? Order the hollandaise sauce on the side and drizzle it on to taste. Breakfast potatoes are ladened with salt and oil, so proceed with caution. You think oatmeal is a heart-healthy choice at brunch? Plain oatmeal is, but not if they add cream or milk, brown sugar, or dried fruit which has as much glycemic load as candy. Ask a lot of questions about how your oatmeal is prepared before diving in.

Whole grain cereal with berries and a splash of low-fat or skim milk for moisture are good options. Waffles, pancakes, umm, need I say major warning – unless you're intentionally going for it? One day I ordered a sweet potato waffle and enjoyed half with a drizzle of all natural maple syrup. As you might imagine, I had been very Good the week prior.

You can eat clean, complex carbs such as whole grains or sweet potatoes earlier in the day or a hearty mixed green salad at lunch (but first read the next chapter about salads dining out). If you order a sandwich at lunch, such as grilled poultry, fish, or even a hamburger, take off the top bread. If given the option, order rye or wheat bread and stay away from white rolls.

Anything that looks good is probably bad. When dining out, it becomes more difficult to know what they use. For instance, sautéed fish is sautéed in what oil? Or omelets, mixed with buttermilk, cream, butter? You never know. It's a crapshoot, but we're having a good time, right? The Marshall Plan lifestyle is not about being unpleasantly rigid, nor causing a scene. It's okay to ask questions and keep substitutions to a minimum – most wait-staff will only get one or two substitutions correct anyway.

Find restaurants that accommodate your culinary needs. If you try a new restaurant and the menu doesn't suit your needs, do the best you can, and never go back.

Quick take-away:
The key to having fun is being fully cognizant when making tasty choices that might not be in the best interest of good health and staying slim. The whole point of Being Good to Be Bad is to have fun. Enjoy!

Salads and the Salad Bar – deception lurks!

Beware of sabotaging yourself with fattening salads.

It seems unfair, but you can add enough bad fat and calories to a salad so that the calorie content exceeds cheesy pizza. Whether ordering from a menu or self-serve at the salad bar, be very selective what you add to your salad plate.

Dark leafy greens are best. Look for descriptions such as "mixed greens," but beware, iceberg lettuce is often mixed in as inexpensive filler. Romaine lettuce looks similar to iceberg but is more nutritious.

Caesar salads are typically made with romaine, but they are one of the unhealthiest choices because Caesar dressing is one of the fattiest dressings. I flip out when I see people ordering Caesar salad as a "diet" meal. Croutons are oil-ladened stale bread, a waste of fat, carbs, and calories. If Caesar salad is the best option available, order it with no dressing, with a side of lemon wedges. (Not delicious, but if you're going to splurge on fat, would it be on a Caesar salad?) You can ask for the Caesar dressing on the side, but in better restaurants they will balk at this because the entire salad is typically tossed in the dressing so the dressing doesn't separate. Pick your poison, I always say. (You might notice I do not care for Caesar salad.)

The other arch-nemesis of salads is the iceberg wedge dripping in blue cheese dressing and sprinkled with bacon bits. It's trendy and it amazes me. Occasionally you'll see it offered over Bibb lettuce, which has more nutrients. If you love it, enjoy.

So far, we just say no to *creamy* dressings such as ranch, Thousand Island, blue cheese, or Caesar, and no croutons. Then there are good add ons gone bad, as in sugar-coated candied nuts, a half a cup of dried raisins or cranberries, and cheese. Even good cheese like feta, mozzarella, goat, or parmesan can sabotage your good intentions if there's too much.

Other adds in moderation: slivered almonds, raw walnuts, cashews, pine nuts, avocado slices, legumes such as garbanzos (a.k.a. chick peas), black or white beans, and black olives. These are all high in good fats, but also high in calories; some is okay, but not a quarter cup of each. If your salad comes heaping with too much of a good thing, move it to the side.

Lean grilled meat, poultry, seafood, or tofu is good; fried is not. Green veggies, artichokes, red peppers, tomatoes, and sun-dried tomatoes are good; shredded cheddar, Swiss, Colby, or pepper jack is not. Stay away from vats of cottage cheese on the salad bar that are most likely 4% fat, not low or fat free. Look for vinaigrette-based dressings. Be cautious with mustard vinaigrettes as they can contain cream or mayo. Sesame oil dressings are okay, but some may have added sugars. And always order dressing on the side; deciding for yourself how much dressing you desire is the smartest choice you can make.

Better choices at a salad bar:

- Romaine lettuce
- Spring Mix
- Spinach
- Cucumbers
- Tomatoes
- Julienne carrots
- Peas
- Broccoli
- Celery
- Cauliflower
- Radishes
- Green or red peppers
- Sugar snap peas
- Mushrooms
- Onions
- Shredded parmesan, Romano, asiago, mozzarella
- Grilled chicken
- Miniature shrimp
- Turkey
- Tofu
- Black olives
- Hard boiled eggs
- Garbanzo beans and other legumes
- Fresh fruit
- Sunflower seeds
- Peanuts
- Slivered almonds
- Vinaigrette dressings
- Italian dressing

- Olive oil
- Balsamic vinegar

Stay away from at a salad bar:
- Iceberg lettuce
- Croutons
- Cottage cheese
- Yogurt
- Shredded cheddar
- Bacon bits
- Diced ham
- Prosciutto
- Dried fruit, raisins, cranberries, dates
- Candied nuts
- Pita chips
- Bread sticks
- Ranch dressing
- Thousand Island dressing
- Caesar dressing
- Canned fruit
- Jello
- Pudding

Quick take-away: Be careful not to eat an excessive amount of calories in a salad - know what you're getting. Aside from the mixed greens, eat everything in moderation.

On the Road

In The Marshall Plan, it's best to never let yourself get too hungry and packing travel snacks is a must do. Eat small meals or snacks throughout the day, for instance at 7am, 10am, noon, 4pm and 7pm. This is the best way to defy the hunger beast. When you're on the road, choices are iffy so that means – pack snacks.

"On the road" means whenever you're on the go, whether it's by planes, trains, or automobiles for long term travel, or just a busy day. I used to stress out when I was forced to sit in all-day group meetings when food choices were challenging. Nightmare scenario: donuts in the morning, deli sandwiches at lunch, candy, cookies, or chips served in the afternoon. If the hosts added a salad, it was often iceberg lettuce, not worth eating. I don't know about you, but I'm a hungry girl, and I gotta eat. The smartest choices aren't always readily on hand unless you pack your travel snacks.

You can buy prepared snacks, but in The Marshall Plan we are trying to eat whole, fresh food. Since that's not always feasible, there are some prepackaged choices that are acceptable as the exception, not the norm.

For the car or in meetings, start with a small travel case for food along with freezer packs if you want to keep things cool. Low-sodium V8 is my number one go to travel snack (with the exception of going through TSA security at the airport.) You get an assortment of vegetables without a lot of calories, fat or sugar, and it fills you up. Raw nuts in a small ziplock travel well, but as we know, nuts add up in calories and fat. If you buy bulk at the market, measure a quarter cup of raw nuts (unsalted roasted in a pinch) of almonds, walnuts, cashews, hazelnuts, or pecans. One-ounce or ounce-and-a-half packages of raw nuts are available in the grocer's bakery aisle. Dry-roasted peanuts are also acceptable, but again, just a quarter cup for the road.

Chopped veggies are a smart choice: baby carrots, celery sticks, and cut red pepper slices all travel well as do cooked (from frozen) edamame in shells, a.k.a. fresh soybeans. Again, mind your portions as they too are heavy on calories and fat grams, albeit good fat.

When staying in hotels, I like to bring healthier snack bars to have on hand for breakfast. This is where reading your labels really matters. You need to identify whether the nutrient count of the bar is a *meal replacement* or a *snack* based on calories, fat, carbs, and sugar. Odwella bars are made from natural ingredients and moderate in fat, sugar, and carbs. I try to eat just half at a time. Other packaged granola or fiber bars are typically high in sugar and carbohydrate, low in protein.

Remember, protein sustains you, fighting off hunger longer. Carbohydrates fill you up temporarily, resulting in feeling sleepy and hungry shortly thereafter.

Low-fat or fat-free yogurts are quick to grab, but really not as healthy a choice as people perceive them to be. By now you know low fat or fat free means added sugar to boost the flavor. The effect is more like a carbohydrate than a protein. Yogurt smoothies and supposedly healthy fruit juices are often two servings per container and really high in sugar. Given the choice between a bag of potato chips or a juice, choose the juice, try drinking half, while making it an exception, not the norm.

Sliced turkey breast or roast beef roll-ups (homemade) are good, but again, go for whole, fresh-sliced deli meats behind the counter versus packaged, sliced meats that are often ladened with fat, sodium, and preservatives, as are other meats like ham, bologna, salami, or anything sliced from a roll. In a pinch, I've packed half a cooked Kashi thin-crust pizza wrapped in tin foil for on-the-go travel food.

Get creative, be prepared, because no matter how different your healthy snacks are, it's going to be better than something you might find in the airport, a fast food chain, or a gas station super-mart. Yes, I've been there, done them all, 'cause when you're hungry, ya gotta eat.

Of course there are the times in life when you're stuck making do with "fast food." Road trips often force us to contemplate less-than-optimal choices. You know, you get to that strip of civilization when you see golden arches, buckets of chicken, talking clowns .... Here I say, pick your poison. If you have a dirty secret desire leftover from childhood for a specific fast food, go for it. Personally, we go for Subway, relatively fresh turkey and assorted veggies. I always have the personal-size bag of Baked Lays, knowing they're not good for me, but I never eat a Subway sandwich without them. Just ain't gonna happen.

Quick take-away:
Be prepared, pack snacks.

CHAPTER 21

A Day in the Life

THROUGHOUT THIS BOOK you've heard about smart choices and Being Good to Be Bad, creating a lifestyle eating regimen that's flexible yet effective in managing your weight to look and feel good.

Just like Baskin Robbins and their 31 Flavors, we all have different tastes, likes, and dislikes. The Marshall Plan has recommendations based on what I like to eat because, well, it's my book! There are many other options out there to help you understand what you can eat to help you Be Good. (It's easy to Be Bad, so no need for help there.) Go to my Facebook page, The Marshall Plan - Being Good to Be Bad, to "like" and share your favorite tactics for Being Good.

Here's a typical Being Good day for me:

Breakfast: Three raw walnuts and eight to 10 ounces of water, followed by one and a half to two cups of 50:50 caf/decaf dark, rich black coffee. Thirty minutes later, a half to a whole cup of assorted fresh fruit topped with chia seeds in summer. Occasionally, a hard boiled egg when traveling.

Morning snack: Lean protein such as tofu cubes with greens, or a quarter avocado or schmear of almond butter on a Scandinavian high fiber, low glycemic bran crisp. In winter, I typically reduce the number of days I eat fruit (0-3) and eat the brans crisps with above mentioned protein options as breakfast, then might have a Greens+ drink mid-morning.

Lunch: Three to four ounces of grilled salmon or occasionally chicken with two servings of mixed green lettuces or steamed or sautéed green vegetables.

Afternoon snack: This is a tough time of day because I'm often hungry and want to eat dinner early. Sometimes I do, depending on the hour. If not, I'll try to stave off hunger with a fresh-pressed green juice or a piece of fruit with almond butter if I hadn't had that in the morning. If I haven't eaten all my lunch protein, I might finish it at this time; or carefully select 10 raw almonds, seven raw cashews, or four Brazil nuts. That's one of the above, not all. And of course, a cup of antioxidant rich Bancha or green tea helps fill the void.

Dinner: Typically vegetarian such as a large bowl of kale salad with a few pine nuts and dried cranberries, or steamed or sautéed vegetables, and sometimes a 100-calorie serving of microwave popcorn, fresh, not packaged.

Evening snack: red raspberry, vanilla, mint, or chocolate mint hot tea.

Quick take-away:
Devise a diverse strategy to Be Good
three or four days a week.

CHAPTER 22

Make Time for Yourself

So MANY PEOPLE are so busy, busy, busy, running to work, taking care of family, even socializing with friends that they don't have time to take care of themselves.

Your good health is of the utmost importance. Without good health, you're down for the count, sidelined, and worse yet, a burden on those you love. Yes, The Marshall Plan is all about having a good time, but the underlying premise is it's up to you to make smart decisions for yourself and for those you love. It's not a perfect world, so when the going gets tough and you want to rip the heads off a package of gummy bears, stop, check in, and ask yourself what's going on.

Refining The Marshall Plan does take time, thought, and effort. You may go to the grocery store more often, or research new recipes or what fruits and vegetables are in season. Find time for a short walk, spend time outside, schedule a night in alone or with people you love.

Hold the same high standards for eating alone as eating with friends and family. Eating is a heartwarming, integral component to life. Don't penalize yourself for eating alone by eating nasty food.

In addition to the foods we eat to feed our bodies, primary foods are the elements that feed our soul. Whether it's reading a good book, listening to music, dancing, or laughing with family and friends, we all need primary foods in our lives. Your primary food might be fulfilling work, whether for income or at home in a garden. It's whatever it is that *makes your heart sing.*

If you're so busy that you do not have time for these things, you're running a rat race that no one is going to win.

Hopefully, throughout this book you keyed in on words like *mindful awareness.* Notice how you feel, whether it's desiring a special food, a particular body image, or an energy level. Be mindful of your surroundings and the people in your life. Notice how you feel.

We are on this earth to live and enjoy a healthy lifestyle, and yes, it's a never-ending battle. None of us will ever master perfect healthy eating all the time, and if we did, wouldn't life be dull?

> *Quick take-away: Love yourself, be good to yourself, and whatever you do, have fun.*

###